Prevention and Treatment of Sports Injuries

Dr. P.L. Karad

KHEL SAHITYA KENDRA
7/26, Ansari Road, Daryaganj,
New Delhi-110002.

Published by:

KHEL SAHITYA KENDRA

7/26, Ansari Road, Darya Ganj, New Delhi-110002

Ph.: (O) 011-43551324, 42564726, 47090343
(M) 9811088729, (Fax) 011-42564726
(Res.) 47091605

E-mail: khelsahitya1@rediffmail.com

Website: www.khelsahitya.com, www.kskpublisher.com

ISBN 978-81-7524-600-3

PRINTED IN INDIA 2026

Printed by:
ASIAN OFFSET PRINTERS
Delhi

Laser Typesetting by:
K.S.K. DTP UNIT, DELHI

CONTENTS

1

SPORTS INJURIES— AN INTRODUCTION

Sports injuries are injuries that occur to athletes in major sporting events. In many cases, these types of injuries are due to overuse of a part of the body when participating in a certain activity. For example, runner's knee is a painful condition generally associated with running, while tennis elbow is a form of repetitive stress injury at the elbow, although it does not often occur with tennis players. Other types of injuries can be caused by a hard contact with something. This can often cause a broken bone or torn ligament or tendon.

Injuries are a common occurrence in professional sports and most teams have a staff of Athletic Trainers and close connections to the medical community. Controversy has arisen at times when teams have made decisions that could threaten a players long-term health for short term gain.

It is inevitable that injuries will always be associated with physical activity and athletics. The risk of injury is much higher in some sports, such as those requiring contact or collision, but is inherent to all athletic activity. Although the majority of athletic injuries are relatively minor, the potential for serious and passible life-threatening injuries is constantly present. The incidence of serious and life-threatening conditions associated with athletic activity has decreased over the last several years as a result of the delineation of causative factors and subsequent rule modifications in many sports and vast improvements and increased sophistication in all facets of sports medicine and athletic training.

In spite of this increased sophistication, there has been an overall increase in the number of athletic injuries; this is primarily the result of an increase in the number of participants, the intensity of modern training techniques and the expansion of athletic activities. Today a wider selection of athletic activities, physical fitness programs and sports are available to a larger cross-section of the population than ever before.

Interest in physical activities and athletics continues to increase and participation in no longer limited to high school, college, amateur, and professional athletes. A greater number of organized athletic programs are available to children in junior high school and upper elementary grades. Youth sports competition, recreational programs, intramural activities, and sports for the handicapped and all age groups are increasing in popularity.

The number of participants in all areas continues to increase dramatically. The development of many women's athletic programs is another factor that has greatly changed the number of sports activities and opportunities for participation. Because of all these developments, there are greater opportunities for persons of all ages to participate in recreational and competitive activities. People are becoming more health and fitness conscious than ever before.

The awareness has produced an increased interest in the benefits of physical fitness. More people than ever before are participating in life-time activities such as walking, jogging, bicycling, swimming, golf, and tennis. People today have more leisure time available as a result of many factors, including shorter work weeks, mechanization, and time-saving devices. Many people are using this additional leisure time to participate in recreational activities requiring some degree of physical exertion.

Whatever the reason for the dramatic increase in the number of participants and activities available, injuries are a reality at every level of participation and in every type of program. Participants in all forms of athletic activity are subjected to many stresses and forces that can result in injury. It is important to remember that injuries to athletes are essentially no different from those suffered by nonathletes.

A sprained ankle can result in the same severity of damage whether it is sustained by a competitive athlete ora week-end jogger. However, the demands in terms of evaluation, treatment, rehabilitation, and return to activity are usually significantly greater for the competitive athlete.

SPORTS MEDICINE

Just as there have been tremendous increases in participation and interest in athletics, there have been corresponding increases in interest, knowledge, and understanding concerning all aspects of the medical management of athletes and athletic injuries.

A new phrase has been coined to describe this vast network of medical management: sports medicine. Sports medicine encompasses all phases of medical concerns relating to the athlete: biomechanical, psychological, nutritional, environmental, pathological, and physiological. The field of sports medicine has seen phenomenal development in recent years, as evidenced by the professional associations designating sports medicine as a speciality, the vast amounts of literature, research, and educational experiences now available, and the number of medical clinics specializing in sports medicine emerging throughout the country.

Sports medicine is a rapidly growing, dynamic field. The knowledge and techniques gained are benefiting not only competitive athletes and the vast legion of fitness buffs but also everyone else involved in athletic and non-athletic activities. Sports medicine includes all medical and para-medical professionals who are concerned with and provide expertise aimed at improving the performance and the health care of athletes. One of the subspecializations of sports medicine is athletic training.

ATHLETIC TRAINING

As a sports medicine subspeciality, athletic training provides a wide array of health care support services for athletes. Athletic training as defined by the National Athletic Trainer's Association is "the art and science of prevention and management of injuries at all levels of athletic activity". The provider of athletic training services is an athletic trainer.

The profession of athletic training and the position of the athletic trainer on the sports medicine team have developed to meet a demand for someone highly skilled in the evaluation, management, and care of athletic injuries. As long as there has been athletics, there has generally been someone designated to manage or care for athletes who become injured.

In the past this position of responsibility was generally filled by a coach, teacher, student, or other interested person. Now many of these positions at the collegiate and professional levels are being filled by a qualified athletic trainer. However, much of the responsibility for the medical care of athletes, particularly at the high-school level, remains with the coach and will continue as such until the need for highly skilled athletic trainers is recognized.

There appears to be a need for an increase in the number and availability of qualified athletic trainers nationally. As compared with other allied health professions, athletic training is quite young. NATA was founded in 1950. The qualifications and requirements to become an athletic trainer have become more stringent over the years. In 1969 a procedure was developed for these institutions offering athletic training curricula to obtain NATA approval.

At that time only two schools were selected that met all requirements for approval. Today there are over 70 schools offering NATA-approved curricula. In 1970 a certifying procedure for athletic trainers was established and has been continually upgraded and improved. To become an athletic trainer a person must possess a college degree that fulfils specific educational and practical requirements. On successful completion of these requirements the candidate must then take a national certifying examination designed to ensure that he or she meets the minimal standards and competencies required to become an athletic trainer.

In addition to obtaining the initial certification, athletic trainers must also earn a designated number of continuing education units to maintain their certified status. Today's athletic trainer is more than just a technician designated to tape ankles, apply bandages, or "rubdown" athletes. Athletic training is becoming more scientific, and athletic trainers are more knowledgeable about the many aspects of health care for athletes. The athletic trainer has become a vital member of the sports medicine team.

In addition to the athletic trainer, this team includes the team physician, coach, and other professionals involved in providing health care for athletes. It is the athletic trainer's responsibility to coordinate the health care services available. In 1982 a role delineation study conducted by the NATA classified the duties or functions of an athletic trainer into six major categories:

(1) prevention

(2) assessment,

(3) treatment, management, and disposition,

(4) rehabilitation,

(5) organization and administration, and

(6) education and counselling of injured athletes.

Each of these areas is important and all are interrelated. The athletic trainer must develop knowledge and competency in each category to provide athletes with optimal medical care. The athletic trainer muse be able to combine medical and scientific information in the areas of anatomy, physiology, kinesiology, psychology, physiology of exercise, health, physics, nutrition, and first aid with a wide array of complex practical skills.

In addition, he or she must also have a sincere interest in athletics and in working with athletes and must possess communication and leadership skills. The athletic trainer is no longer a "jack of all trades, master of none". He or she is a professional who must be proficient in many varied skills.

ASSESSMENT

Athletic trainers must possess a high level of proficiency in assessment skills to accurately recognize and evaluate the nature and severity of an athletic injury. Athletic trainers are normally at the location or playing field where an injury occurs and will have to handle the emergency care. They must be able to recognize and deal with such conditions as severe head or spine injuries, haemorrhaging, shock, heat illness, or choking.

Athletic trainers must be prepared to administer cardiopulmonary resuscitation, apply emergency splinting, or supervise the transportation of an injured athlete. The athletic injury assessment process is based on a scientific method that involves:

(a) recognition and statement of the problem,

(b) creation and testing of hypotheses to solve the solve the problem,

(c) collection of data about the problem.

An athletic trainer's initial assessment creates the foundation or data base for the ensuing procedures. It begins with the collection of data related to the injury through the systematic steps of history, observation, palpation, and stress manoeuvres. From the data collected, the athletic trainer must determine and initiate the appropriate course of action. This includes emergency medical care, follow-up treatment procedures, transportation, medical referral, rehabilitation strategies, or return to athletic activity.

Once action has been taken, the athletic trainer must continually evaluate the results of this action. Is the athletic getting better or worse? Why? What can be done to improve or enhance the athlete's recovery? The athletic trainer should then modify or adjust the plan of action accordingly. Assessment and reassessment are going processes in athletic training.

REHABILITATION

Rehabilitation is the restoration of normal form and function after an injury. Athletic rehabilitation is the reconditioning of an injured athlete to his or her highest level of function in the shortest possible time. This level of function is generally higher than that of a nonathlete. Athletic trainers must be skilled in developing programs to effectively rehabilitate an athlete in a minimal amount of time.

Depending upon the nature and the conditions surrounding the injury, rehabilitation requires a progressive, systematic program that develops range of motion, muscular strength and endurance, coordinated movements, functional activities, and circulorespirator endurance. Although each of these phases overlap, maximal development of any phases requires prior development of the preceding phase. During rehabilitation there should be repeated assessment techniques performed to evaluate progress and indicate appropriate follow-up care.

PREVENTION

The best method of managing and caring for athletic injuries is to prevent them from occurring; thus much of the athletic trainer's time and effort is devoted to preventing injuries. Numerous factors briefly discussed in this section are important in the prevention of athletic injuries. A thorough pre-participation evaluation does not guarantee that an athlete will participate injury free but it does firm that there is no discernible clinical reason to preclude participation. Proper conditioning is the preventing medicine of athletics.

Athletic trainers often work in conjunction with coaches in establishing pre-season, in-season, and post-season conditioning programs. Another facet of athletic injury prevention in which the athletic trainer is involved is the selection, fitting, and maintenance of protective equipment. An athletic trainer may also be responsible for checking the safety of facilities and apparatus required for athletic activity. More familiar preventive tasks performed by athletic trainers include the application of protective taping, padding, bandaging, braces, and other devices.

Athletic trainers must also constantly observe their athletes. If recognized early, minor problems can often be treated with minimal inconvenience to the athlete and no significant decrease in performance. Early recognition and effective treatment prevent most minor injuries from becoming more severe and disabling. An injury that is properly recognized and managed effectively generally does not become more severe, and the potential for reinjury is less.

In addition, athletic trainers are often asked to counsel athletes and coaches in the areas of diet, rest, and sanitation.

MANAGEMENT AND TREATMENT

Athletic trainers must be skilled in various management and treatment procedures. These include:

(1) administering immediate first aid,

(2) providing therapy to promote healing, and recovery,

(3) applying protective techniques to support and protect an injured area, and

(4) referring an injured athlete for other medical assistance when necessary.

Athletic trainers can have a dramatic effect on the overall recovery of an injured athlete by the proper use of treatment procedures. The goal is to return the injured athlete to activity as soon as possible without risking further injury. The treatment of an athletic injury is a three-step process:

(1) examination of the signs and symptoms,

(2) application of treatment routines, and

(3) assessment of the effects of these techniques on the signs and symptoms of the injury.

This cycle continues throughout the treatment process; that is, assessment, treatment, and reassessment. If an athlete is no return optimum physical activity in a minimal amount of time, there can be no delay in an accurate assessment and a properly instituted treatment program.

ORGANISATION AND ADMINISTRATION

Often overlooked aspects of an athletic trainer's responsibilities are the organization and administration of the athletic training program, Athletic trainers must plan, organize, evaluate, and implement procedures and policies necessary to provide their athletes with the most effective health care available.

To aid in efficient health care delivery, athletic trainers must maintain accurate and detailed records to document injuries and treatments and other services rendered to the athletes under their care. Selecting, purchasing, maintaining, and instructing others in the use of equipment and supplies necessary for operation of a training room are also the athletic trainer's responsibilities.

EDUCATION AND COUNSELLING

The last function of an athletic trainer to be discussed is the role of education and counsellor to the athlete and student athletic trainer. Athletic trainers need to have the skill and knowledge necessary to instruct students in the competencies required to become professional athletic trainers.

This responsibility requires that the athletic trainer keep abreast of current sports medicine issues and also be able to convey this information to others. Another facet of education and counselling skills required is the athletic trainer's ability to recognize situations requiring consultation with other health care professionals regarding an athlete's social or personal problem. This involves skill in assessing an athlete's need for professional consultation and referral of the athlete to the appropriate professional.

To be effective communication skills. These communication skills enable the athletic trainer to interact with athletes, parents, coaches, administrators, physicians and other professionals concerning various health-related topics. To summarize, athletic trainer must develop knowledge and competency in each of these duties or functions to provide optimal medical care to athletes. Note that assessment or evaluation skills are listed and discussed under each of these categories. Athletic injury assessment is a necessary and extremely important skill for anyone who has medical responsibilities for athletes.

CLASSIFICATION

Sports injuries can be broadly classified as either traumatic or overuse injuries. Traumatic injuries account for most injuries in contact sports such as Football, Rugby, Australian rules football, Gaelic football and American football because of the dynamic and high collision nature of these sports. These injuries range from bruises and muscle strains, to fractures and head injuries.

A bruise or contusion is damage to small blood vessels which causes bleeding within the tissues. A muscle strain is a small tear of muscle fibers and a ligament sprain is a small tear of ligament tissue. The body's response to these sports injuries is the same in the initial five day period immediately following the traumatic incident - inflammation.

SIGNS AND SYMPTOMS

Inflammation is characterized by pain, localized swelling, heat, redness and a loss of function.

MECHANISM

All of these traumatic injuries cause damage to the cells that make up the soft tissues. The dead and damaged cells release chemicals, which initiate an inflammatory response. Small blood vessels are damaged and opened up, producing bleeding within the tissue. In the body's normal reaction, a small blood clot is formed in order to stop this bleeding and from this clot special cells (called fibroblasts) begin the healing process by laying down scar tissue.

The inflammatory stage is therefore the first phase of healing. However, too much of an inflammatory response in the early stage can mean that the healing process takes longer and a return to activity is delayed. The sports injury treatments are intended to minimize the inflammatory phase of an injury, so that the overall healing process is accelerated. intrinsic and extrinsic factors

PREVENTION

A comprehensive warm-up programme has been found to decrease injuries in soccer. Many athletes will partake in HGH Treatment for Athletic Enhancement as a way to prevent injuries.

Treatment

Sports injuries can be treated and managed by using the P.R.I.C.E.R... DR. ABC and T.O.T.A.P.S regimes:

P - Protect

R - Rest

I - Ice

C - Compression

E - Elevation

R - Referral

D - Danger

R - Response

A - Airway

B - Breathing

C. - Circulation

T - Talk

O - Observe

T - Touch

A - Active movement

P - Passive movement

S - Skills test

The inflammatory stage typically lasts around 5 days and all treatment during this time is designed to address the cardinal signs of inflammation – pain, swelling, redness, heat and a loss of function.

Kinesiology tape, also known as elastic therapeutic tape, is used in therapy to treat injuries and relax overused muscles, and in rehabilitation to facilitate underused muscles. The wave pattern found on the tape's adhesive has a lifting effect on the skin which can reduce swelling and inflammation by improving circulation and reduce pain by taking pressure off pain receptors. Today Kinesiology tape is accepted by medical practitioners and athletes in Japan, the United States, Europe, South America, Australia, and other Asian countries. Kinesiology tape is just starting to be available to average consumers for the first time in 2009.

Compression sportswear is becoming very popular with both professional and amateur athletes. These garments are thought to both reduce the risk of muscle injury and speed up muscle recovery.

Portable Mild Hyperbaric Chamber 40" diameterAlthough not proven some professional athletes use hyperbaric chambers to speed healing. Hines Ward of the Steelers sent his personal hyperbaric chamber,(similar to the one pictured), to his hotel to sleep in believing it would help heal his sprained medial collateral ligament he suffered in their playoff win against the Ravens. Hines went on to play in Super Bowl

XLIII.

Knee Injuries and Recovery

The knee is a core tool for an athlete; it allows football and basketball players to run, cut, and jump. Baseball players use their knees to push off when they throw. The flexibility and rotational ability of a knee is what helps make some tennis players superstars. It's difficult to return to competitive athletics after any serious injury, but knee injuries takes a lot longer to get over and often end a career. While having a good physical rehab process is very important, the athlete's ability to overcome the mental hurdles that are created with a knee injury will determine whether or not he will be the same player that he was before the injury.

The words "it's an ACL" strike fear in the heart of an athlete. The immediate mental translation is will I ever play again and if I do play will I ever be as good? Why do knee injuries cause so much fear in competitive athletes? According to the Brown University Biology and Medicine Web site, athletes in contact sports are 10 times more likely to have a serious knee injury than in non-contact sports, with knee injuries accounting for approximately a quarter of the injuries and generally taking two to three times longer to recovery than injuries to other parts of the body Knee injuries are also increasing, "over the last 15 years, ankle sprains have decreased by 86% and tibia fractures by 88%, but knee ligament injuries have increased by 172%".

What cause knee injuries and what is the prognosis for total rehabilitation? Leg bones are connected to the kneecap by four strong ligaments: Anterior Cruciate Ligament (ACL), Lateral Collateral Ligament (LCL), Medial Collateral Ligament (MCL), and Posterior Cruciate

Ligament (PCL). The ACL provides stability and controls stress across the kneecap and keeps the knee from rotating too much or moving too far forward. Around 60% of ligament tears are ACL, most occurring in basketball, skiing, football and soccer. When an ACL tears it unravels like a rope and will not heal on its own. For competitive athletes treatment is almost always surgery. It normally takes 6 to 9 months to recovery from an ACL reconstruction surgery, at which point most athletes had returned to between 80% and 100% of their full level of previous play with about 90% returning to competition. After the first ACL injury, there is a 5 to 15% risk of repeated injury. MCL and LCL ligament tears are less frequent then ACL injuries accounting for about 25% with LCL injury being much less frequent than MCL injuries. MCL injuries are normally caused when a significant force is applied to the side of the knee while the lower leg is held in a fixed position. The MCL is the only ligament that has enough of a blood supply to heal partial tears without surgery PCL injuries account for between 3% and 20% of all tears. Most often the cause is a blow to a bent leg. Because of the type of blow, PCL tears are often accompanied by ACL tears. While conservative treatment is still controversial in some sports for both PCL and MCL tears, it has proven to be as effective in returning an athlete back to his playing condition as has surgery.

Why or why not surgery? If an athlete wants to play competitively ACL tears require reconstructive surgery. During surgery the old ACL is removed, a graft from the patellar tendon or the hamstring is prepared, holes are drilled in the tibia and femur and the graft is attached with screws to the bones. Now the tough part begins, surgery is followed by 6 to 9 months of rehabilitation.

This rehabilitation is crucial to strengthen the areas surrounding the graft so that it does not fail. Athletes may accept that injuries are part of their lives and may know how to deal with physical rehabilitation, but few are prepared for the emotional pain, fear and anger that also result from injury. Athletes are used to being part of a team. When they are injured they are suddenly on their own. Their teammates will continue on but they now have a new job, physical and emotional rehabilitation of their bodies and much of the work will have to be accomplished on their own. In Sidelines, Psyched Up or Psyched Out? David Doermann describes a University of Utah pamphlet that is given to all student athletes to help them understand what to expect if they are injured. It describes the emotional process that happens when someone is injured as similar to the five stages of grief The first stage is denial. Athletes by their very nature believe that they are superior physically and therefore do not accept the fact they can be injured. When an athlete realizes an injury is real his reaction may be to isolate and blame himself. Denial is followed by anger, particularly at himself for allowing the injury to occur. During the third stage the athlete tries to make bargains with coaches, trainers or God, such as if I spend 2 hours walking every day I can play again in 2 months.

Very often these bargains are unreasonable dreams. The competitive athlete will now move to a period of depression, feeling sorry for themselves, withdrawing or simply giving up. This stage particularly can put an athlete's rehab off track. To be successful an athlete must finally get to the acceptance stage when he realizes that the only way to handle the injury is to focus on his physical rehab which could result in returning to competition. The factors that contribute the most to helping an athlete reach psychological acceptance and recovery are education, social support, psychological skill training and goal setting; traits that many athletes use in their pre-injury training.

Understanding an injury and their reaction to it helps athletes cope with the problems that naturally arrive along with the injury. Support and understanding of team mates, family and friends can also be a critical factor in recovery. Knowing and understanding how others have coped gives athletes mechanisms for starting to construct their own recoveries. While having social support that listens and appreciates the seriousness of an injury is necessary, too much sympathy from family or friends can impair the athlete's acceptance level which can slow or derail the recovery process.

Rehabilitation

Rehabilitation is the restoration of normal form and function after an injury. Athletic rehabilitation is the reconditioning of an injured athlete to his or her highest level of function in the shortest possible time. This level of function is generally higher than that of a nonathlete. Athletic trainers must be skilled in developing programs to effectively rehabilitate an athlete in a minimal amount of time.

Depending upon the nature and the conditions surrounding the injury, rehabilitation requires a progressive, systematic program that develops range of motion, muscular strength and endurance, coordinated movements, functional activities, and circulorespirator endurance. Although each of these phases overlap, maximal development of any phases requires prior development of the preceding phase. During rehabilitation there should be repeated assessment techniques performed to evaluate progress and indicate appropriate follow-up care.

Prevention

The best method of managing and caring for athletic injuries is to prevent them from occurring; thus much of the athletic trainer's time and effort is devoted to preventing injuries. Numerous factors briefly discussed in this section are important in the prevention of athletic injuries. A thorough pre-participation evaluation does not guarantee that an athlete will participate injury free but it does firm that there is no discernible clinical reason to preclude participation. Proper conditioning is the preventing medicine of athletics.

Athletic trainers often work in conjunction with coaches in establishing pre-season, in-season, and post-season conditioning programs. Another facet of athletic injury prevention in which the athletic trainer is involved is the selection, fitting, and maintenance of protective equipment. An athletic trainer may also be responsible for checking the safety of facilities and apparatus required for athletic activity. More familiar preventive tasks performed by athletic trainers include the application of protective taping, padding, bandaging, braces, and other devices.

Athletic trainers must also constantly observe their athletes. If recognized early, minor problems can often be treated with minimal inconvenience to the athlete and no significant decrease in performance. Early recognition and effective treatment prevent most minor injuries from becoming more severe and disabling. An injury that is properly recognized and managed effectively generally does not become more severe, and the potential for reinjury is less.

In addition, athletic trainers are often asked to counsel athletes and coaches in the areas of diet, rest, and sanitation.

Management and Treatment

Athletic trainers must be skilled in various management and treatment procedures. These include:

(1) administering immediate first aid,

(2) providing therapy to promote healing, and recovery,

(3) applying protective techniques to support and protect an injured area, and

(4) referring an injured athlete for other medical assistance when necessary.

Athletic trainers can have a dramatic effect on the overall recovery of an injured athlete by the proper use of treatment procedures. The goal is to return the injured athlete to activity as soon as possible without risking further injury. The treatment of an athletic injury is a three-step process:

(1) examination of the signs and symptoms,

(2) application of treatment routines, and

(3) assessment of the effects of these techniques on the signs and symptoms of the injury.

This cycle continues throughout the treatment process; that is, assessment, treatment, and reassessment. If an athlete is no return optimum physical activity in a minimal amount of time, there can be no delay in an accurate assessment and a properly instituted treatment program.

2

ADMINISTRATION OF SPORTS INJURIES

Administration of sports injury requires substantially more than 'treatment' of an injured area. Patients need advice on a number of other aspects, including maintenance of overall fitness during recovery, and require a suitable prognosis. If physical treatment is desirable it is necessary to have some knowledge of therapeutic modalities, and preferably a sound professional working relationship with the therapist of choice. It is erroneous to assume automatically that ice and ultrasound, for instance, cure all soft tissue lesions; more critical evaluation of the options is required before prescribing specific therapeutic regimes. A good physical therapist needs, above all else, a diagnosis, following which he/she will probably have more experience in the usefulness of modalities such as effleurage, friction massage, laser therapy, etc. than the referring practitioner. However, it is incumbent upon the referring doctor to offer guidance, and thereby encourage suitable feedback of information on patients' progress.

Depending on the type, severity, and duration of the injury, it may be necessary for the patient to progress from the therapy room to the rehabilitation area, where progressive strengthening exercises and flexibility exercises may be performed. Isotonic, isometric, and isokinetic exercises all have their place; they hold to combined with setal stretching schedules. With a greater availability of gymnasia and health clubs, in which sophisticated equipment such as the Nautilus range is commonly available for both training and rehabilitation, it is increasingly important for progress to be monitored by the practitioner and for prescriptive exercises to be specific to both the injury and the sport. It is often forget that stretching exercises which are primarily performed for specific muscle groups may impose stresses on other parts of the body—this is particularly relevant to the prevention of spinal injury during the rehabilitation of an injured limb.

Liaison with the coach or trainer should be considered to be an important aspect of both assessment and management. The coaches of athletes, particularly those in the younger age groups with considerable attitude, may well be ale to furnish useful information regarding the cause of injury which has not otherwise been disclose; conversely they need guidance on the reduction of specific forms of stress during the subsequent resumption of training. Occasions frequently arise when a telephone call to the coach of an up-and-coming tennis starlet, for instance, reveals the existence of normal biomechanical stress associated with faulty serving technique. Hyperextention of the spine on tennis service or excessive forearm rotation on the forehand are not uncommon. Unless such information is presented to the physician, and flawed technique identified and corrected, recurrence of injury is to be expected.

Overall, the patient needs reassurance, whenever possible, regarding he likelihood of a satisfactory outcome, as his worst fears are not always overly expressed. The parents of a adolescent with Osgood-Schlatter's disease often need a positive statement that the 'lump' is not a tumour, and likewise the patient with a thigh swelling from a rectus femoris tear. In this branch of medicine, in which the frustration of injury is often compounded by a psychological 'low' secondary to inactivity, sympathetic understanding is required. Too many patients inappropriately receive a bland prescription for absolute rest, or an unhelpful reaction such as, 'I am not surprise that you have leg pain if you run seventy miles a week.' Patients, quite rightly, expect advice for injuries that have occurred in an era when recreation and sport are encouraged, not least by government-backed 'Sport for All' and 'Exercise for Health' campaigns. The abrogation by some members of the medical profession of their responsibility to provide a caring service on the grounds that sports injuries are 'self-induced' is quite intolerable. Despite the reluctance of central government to release funding for Sports Injury Clinics or for postgraduate medical education in sports medicine, increasing expectations on the part of patients are likely to be a major stimulus to the development of a greater awareness of the need for the advancement of sports medicine within the medical profession. It is hoped that funds from the National Lottery will be a further stimulus to the development of regional centres of excellence in Sports Medicine. However, doctors of first contact will take the brunt of an increasing workload.

Judgement

A basic knowledge of the biomechanical forces involved in 'normal' participation in specific sports is required. Track athletes run anti-clockwise both in their events ad during training, so that asymmetrical forces are continually being applied to their lower limbs in particular. Javelin throwers may have an overhead style, or end to sling, in which case different forces are applied to their shoulders and elbows. Tennis players may use a single-or a two-handed backhand, imposing different stresses upon the trunk and upper limbs, and so on. Numerous examples are give throughout the text. These technical factors are particularly relevant when considering overuse injury.

An assessment of joint mobility some distance away from the site of injury is also included in the categorization of relevant aetiological factors. A squash player with a limited range of hip rotation, owing to early degenerative disease, may develop low back pain when excessive rotational stress is repeatedly transferred to the lumbar spine. Weakness or tightness of one group of muscles acting about a joint may similarly result in injury elseback problems, or for muscle injury in compensating muscle groups.

These are simply a few of the factors that require identification for full assessment of the nature of the injury. Training schedules, behavioural tendencies, particularly the behavioural aspects of pain perception, individual motivation, and ambition also need study. Although 'holistic' medicine enjoys much popularity at the moment, it has surely always been incumbent upon medical practitioners to develop a breath of vision which includes every patient—a facet of their skills that they are trained in from the first weeks of the clinical curriculum in medical school. Sports injuries need no less perspicacity than other illnesses that are recognizably 'stress' related. When injuries in children are considered, the interrelationship between ambition on the part of the patient, parents, coaches, and teachers becomes even more important.

The history given by he patient is often revealing. When injury is acute, particularly when extrinsic forces are involved, the direction of the externally applied forces should be established if possible. When injury is of a more chronic nature the history is quite different, as exemplified by the phases of discomfort experienced during he development of tendinitis:

(a) discomfort after activity;

(b) discomfort worsening during activity, associated with functional impairment;

(c) discomfort during the initiation of activity, subsequently improving during further activity, and worsening afterwards;

(d) discomfort sufficient effectively to prevent activity.

Following he extraction of a symptom history and relevant background information, the establishment of a satisfactory diagnosis requires the application to the musculoskeletal system of examination techniques which previously may not have been extensively used by the majority of doctors. An appreciation must be gained of the importance of an examination routine that is founded upon sound orthopaedic principles, so that an assessment of function may be made. The moving parts require clinical appraisal according to the following code.

(i) Active movements.

(ii) Neurological and vascular examination.

(iii) Resisted—i.e. isometric—muscle contraction.

(iv) Observation.

(v) Passive movements.

(vi) Palpation.

The passive movements offer information on joint function and the integrity of the articular structures, and may be further subdivided into

(a) range of motion

(b) 'joint play'

(c) stress testing for ligamentous competency.

The only compromise to this orthopaedic medical system of examination should be when, as a result of a history of acute trauma and the disposition of the patient or of the injured area, a fracture is suspected: gentle handling of the injured site may be followed by early X-ray, prior to more extensive examination procedures if appropriate.

Further investigations such as X-rays, arthrography, ultrasound scans, bone scans, CT scans, MRI scans, hematology, etc., should be considered where relevant. Full assessment relies on an understanding that, just as there is a wider range of ECG changes in an athlete tan in he non-sporting population, so 'abnormal' findings, such as are seen in X-rays of 'footballer's ankle' or on bone scans of long-distance runners termed increased a uptake in the bones of the owner limbs are simply a manifestation of recurrent physical stress. Interpretation must therefore by made wit due care.

Features of Soft Tissue Breakdown and Repair

(i) Remodelling

The process of collagen maturation continues for some weeks and months thereafter. Collagen turnover is maximal in the early stages, when linear thickening may be palpable. The orderly deposition of maturing fibres is presumably dependent upon numerous factors, to least of which are the mechanical stresses to which they are subjected. Initial deposition may e somewhat haphazard, yet improved—that is, fibers are laid down in parallel—if the healing tissue is subjected to gentle stress, and is allowed to undergo a restricted amount of normal function. Noyes et al, have demonstrated the increase in wound strength related to mobilization rather than immobilization. Thus early gentle mobilization after connective tissue injury is desirable, and immobilization techniques are best eschewed unless absolutely necessary.

(ii) Acute inflammatory phase

When injury is sustained to the soft tissues, whether as a result of acute trauma or of repeated microtrauma, localized cellular damage results. In the early inflammatory phase chemotactic agents are released from platelets and mast cells. These agents stimulate the migration of polymorphs and monocytes. Degenerative enzymes are released from a range of inflammatory cells. The concentration of the chemotactic agents appears to be dependent, in part, upon a raised intracellular level of calcium ions. Vasodilation and increased capillary permeability occur, mediated. Interstitial oedema and frank bleeding into the tissues from the larger blood vessels are features of this early phase. During the inflammatory phase over the next few days, in the continued presence of macrophages, further chemotactic factors are released from within their granules: such factors stimulate the development of undifferentiated connective tissue cells into fibroblasts and endothelial and other mature cells.

If sufficiently severe, the inflammatory phase is responsible for the clinical features of erythema, heat, pain, crepitus, swelling, and dysfunction. The physical modalities of treatment help alleviate the symptoms and the extent of the inflammatory process. Prostaglandin synthesis is inhibited by non-steroidal anti-inflammatory drugs. Although it is conventional to think in terms of 'anti-inflammatory' treatment for acute soft tissue injury, the inflammatory phase is nevertheless essential to normal repair. Therefore modalities such as ultrasound may more accurately be considered to be 'pro-inflammatory' by stimulating mast cell activity, and accelerating the normal repair process. In chronic inflammatory conditions, however, it is more appropriate to remove the inflammatory stimulus before the use of specific therapeutic modalities. However, despite relative, or even 'complete', rest, some chronic inflammatory conditions appear to be self-perpetuating. Stress reduction may then need to be combined with the more powerful anti-inflammatory activity of the injectable corticosteriods.

(iii) Proliferative phase

Within a few days of injury the proliferative phase commences, thereby overlapping the late inflammatory phase. Fibroblasts form a connective tissue matrix and endothelial cells develop into blood vessels; the resulting ugly cellular and vascularized tissue is known as granulation tissue. It is essential at this stage that the collagenous matrix is allowed to proceed to relative maturity without the imposition of excessive stress. In more chronic conditions, particularly in poorly vascularized tissue such as tendons, it may be useful to stimulate therapeutically he development of endothelial cells into capillaries. Extensive tissue destruction from the inflammatory phase or excessive tibrosis may sometimes develop, for example in chronic subacromial bursitis and Achilles peritendinitis, thereby creating the risk of permanent dysfunction.

Classification

Injuries can be classified according to their nature or aetiology into

(1) overuse

(2) trauma

1. Overuse

When describing the nature of overuse injury to patients an analogy may be useful. Non-biological materials. Such as aeroplane wings, have a fixed stress point, and if they are subjected to a defined number of flights fatigue fracture will inevitably result. Biological materials ad organisms, on the other hand, may, with carefully graded incremental increases in stress, withstand the most enormous loads—for instance the reputed forces as high as ten times body-weight in the Achilles tendon during running. Nevertheless if the application of submaximal stress has not been carefully graded, or there are adverse biomechanical stress factors, subsequent breakdown of the tissues results in stress or overuse injury. This may occur in any tissue, from bone to bursa.

Whatever the cause or type of injury sustained, the response of the tissue is the development of inflammation. In some rheumatological conditions the causative factor is known: bacteria, uric acid, and pyrophosphate crystals for instance. Tissuc breakdown products resulting from repeated microtrauma are probably responsiblc for inflammation in overuse injury.

Trauma Traumatic incidents occur suddenly, an can be considered to be direct or indirect in type. Examplcs of the former are direct blows to te body, for instance from the force of a cricket ball or as the result of an opponent's punch in boxing, or direct confrontations with immovable forces, for example falling heavily to the ground. Injury to either the hard or soft tissues may occur, and may present to the attendant medical officer, general practitioner, or traumatologist in the local Accident and Emergency Department. In-depth analysis of fractures will generally not be undertaken in this book, though emphasis will be placed upon their recognition. Certain fractures--for example those to the wrist and hand—will be given further consideration, as early diagnosis and appropriate management. If necessary by referral for an expert opinion, are often required for good functional results.

Indirect, trauma indicates the application of stress some distance from the site of injury, or not involving direct body contact. The tissues involved may be muscular, tendinous, ligamentous, osseous, or cartilaginous. The latter may be further osseous, or cartilaginous. The latter may be further divided into injuries to articular cartilage, or to fibro and hyaline cartilage, for example intervertebral injury.

Tissue Injury

Ligament

Ligament are composed primarily of bundles of collagen, demonstrating a greater 'weave' pattern than tendons which have a similar structure. Ligaments are the 'static' stabilizers of joints, though the presence of elastin allows some elongation under stress. At a certain stress level—yield point—deformation of collagen fibres becomes excessive, with the formation of microtears and the loss of previous resting length. Frank rupture then occurs. Assessment of ligamentous competence is by stress testing in various positions of the joint. The clinical aspects of ligament injuries, as they are often inadequately assessed and therefore commonly mismanaged. Important factors to appreciate following ligament injury are as follows.

(i) The proprioceptive reflex is usually profoundly deranged as a result of disturbance to or disruption of the articular mechanoreceptors found in the joint cupules and ligaments. Specific rehabilitative exercises are required for restoration of function.

(ii) Intracapsular bleeding take place—for instance, rupture of the anterior cruciate ligament, in which situation the resulting hemarthrosis must be recognized and dealt with by aspiration or washing out so as to reduce the severely irritating effect of blood on the synovium. A hemarthrosis may be suspected when a joint wells substantially within a couple of hours of the injury. A serious effusion, on the other hand, normally takes twenty-four hours to arise, and thus is usually recognized by the patient the following day. A hemarthrosis may develop in any joint; beneficial results of aspiration may be expected in such joints as the ankle, the elbow, and the interphalangeal joint of the hallux, as well as the knee. The immediate injection steroid in appropriate dosage, once fracture or osteochondra injury has been excluded, should be considered. For aspiration it is essential to have a sound knowledge of topical anatomy.

(iii) Capsular disruption may occur, resulting in substantial soft-tissue bleeding and oedema.

(iv) Joint stability is created by ligaments and muscles. A significant degree of ligament rupture may give rise to mechanical instability, incurring the risk of permanent functional instability—for example, ankle and knee ligament tears. Ligament injuries can be divided into three grades:

(a) partial tear, in which some degree of joint laxity secondary to ligamentous insufficiency is recognized:

(b) completely tear, in which dislocation or substantial disruption of the joint occur.

(c) sprain, in which there is no macroscopic

discontinuity;

(v) Disorganization of the parallel alignment of collagen fibres and bundles in ligaments occurs after immobilization.

(vi) The proprioceptive reflex is usually profoundly deranged as a result of disturbance to or disruption of the articular mechanoreceptors fond in the joint capsules and ligaments. Specific rehabilitative exercises are required for restoration of function.

Cartilage

The articular surfaces of joints with a wide range of movement are composed of hyaline cartilage. Intervertebral discs and intra-articular menisci contain fibrocartilage. Chondral injury or osteochondral injury occurs after jarring or compression. Common sites are the ankle, knee, and elbow. There may be a history of acute trauma when an initial hemarthrosis is followed by recurrent pain and swelling as one articular surface impinges on another; there is a further possibility of loose body formation resulting in temporary locking of the joint. An acute carrying injury to the ankle may cause a osteochondral fracture of the dome of the talus. During patella dislocation an osteochondral fracture involving the posterior surface of the patella is to be expected. Although there is dispute over the aetiology of osteochondritis dissecans, this condition, which commonly occurs in the teenager, may be due to recurrent compression trauma resulting in osteochondral fragmentation and separation. Frequent compression secondary to valgus strain is responsible for osteochondritis of the capitellum at the elbow in gymnasts and baseball pitchers.

Articular cartilage is nourished by synovial fluid, which appears to be dependent upon joint motion for normal function. Degenerative changes, including erosions, may be seen in articular cartilage following prolonged immobilization.

Prolapse of an intervertebral disc occurs when the gelatinous nucleus pulposus herniates through a ruptured annulus. Previous stress changes will probably have already occurred at the disc, manifesting as small radial tears, so that the provocative traumatic incident may be apparently trivial or even not recorded at all.

The menisci which are present in other joints—for instance, the acromioclavicular and radiocarpal joints—may also be deranged by trauma.

Bone

The application of force to a joint or limbs may give rise to osseous injury, either at the joint of impact or some distance away hence the fractures that occur around the ankle on rotating the leg on a fixed foot, fracture of te scaphoid on forced dorsiflexion of the wrist, and fracture of the clavicle on falling on the outstretched hand. Although management of major fractures lies within the province of the orthopaedic surgeon, the simpler fractures, often not requiring fixation, are described in the present study. Guidance is also offered concerning the timely referral of injuries such as hand fractures, which requires particularly good functional results.

In children fractures often accurate the epiphyseal plate, which is responsible for longitudinal growth of the bone, and is weaker than both ligaments ad tendons. Of course, the presence of angulation suggests the presence of a fracture, possibly epiphyseal, and indicates the need for referral; the possibility of epiphyseal fracture should also be considered in the absence of significant deformity when a dislocation or even a sprain is diagnosed. Fractures involving the epiphyseal plate have been categorized into five types of Saltër and Harris. Separations usually heal satisfactorily unless there is vascular disturbance. Fractures across the plate need careful assessment by an orthopaedic surgeon, as premature fusion and a shortened limb may result.

Traction injuries, sometimes termed traction osteochondroses, occur at the apophyses. These are a particularly common type of stress injury in the adolescent—for instance, at he tibial tubercle and oscalcis: they result from overactivity. At some sites around the pelvis—for example, the anterior superior iliac spine, the anterior inferior iliac spine, the lesser trochanter, and the ischial tuberosity—the injury to the apophysis may be due to acute trauma. Fracture separation of the apopysis takes place, and the injury behaves effectively as an acute muscle tear, which is its counterpart in the adult. Rarely, a similar injury occurs at the shoulder, for example avulsion of the subscapularis attachment to the lesser tuberosity.

Tendon

Tendons connect muscle to bone, and are composed of blocks of collagen and elastin. These collagen fibres are highly ordered; their function is to withstand the distractive force associated with muscle contraction. Tendon is able to withstand approximately half the tensile strength of cortical bone, and twice the tensile strength of the associated muscle. The basic pathophysiological cause for breakdown is the repetitive application of tensile forces beyond the biomechanical yield strength of the tendon. Although many tendinoplasties are the result of oversue, some injuries, such as complete or partial rupture, are acute. Even so an acute-on-chronic situation may arise. It is recognized that middle-aged sedentary males are at risk of rupturing their Achilles tendons when undertaking a sudden or unexpected burst of running; it is not always so readily appreciated that chronic stress in the experienced athlete may so undermine the tensile properties of tendon as to result in a likelihood of rupture. Sudden contraction of an already stretched musculotendinous until may be the final provocative stress. The tensile strength of tendons may also be reduced by steroid injections, which should never be given into weightbearing tendons.

Since the musculotendinous unit acts as a united contractile structure the clinical examination procedures in tendon injury are the same as for muscle injury., Although tendon may heal with conservative measures, there are circumstances when a surgical approach is desirable, not least to allow more accurate approximation of the ruptured ends by evacuation of hemorrhage or granulomatous tissue.

Enthesitis is the term applied to a lesion that occurs at an enthesis—i.e. the teno-osseous junction. Examples of enthesopathies are lateral epicondylitis, chronic adductor longus strain, and patella tendinitis.

A tendinitis is normally secondary to oversue. It may occur in a tendon that is essentially healthy in other respects, or in one in which a central or focal degenerative process has taken place. Repetitive submaximal loading leads to recurrent microtrauma in the presence of a poor blood supply. Occasionally calcium hydroxy-apatite crystals are deposited in a degenerative tendon: he resulting calcific tendinitis may be acutely painful.

If the tendon has a sheath, a tenosynovitis may result from overuse: occasionally this may be crepitating, as in intersection syndrome of the forearm. If the tendon has a paratenon, paratendintis—for example Achilles paratendinitis—may develop secondary to an underlying tendinitis, or be caused primarily by friction from extrinsic causes. A complication is the development of chronic paratendinitis, when the paratenon becomes progressively thickened, and may require surgical excision.

Joint

The capsular pattern

The soft tissue components of a joint are the synovium and capsule. When a joint is injured or inflamed from whatever cause its movements are restricted, initially from involuntary muscle spasms, in a capsular pattern. Capsular patterns vary from one joint to another, though are identical from one person to another, and are described in the present study. The same pattern is produced by different provocative stresses—for example, synovial irritation from a hemarthrosis, rheumatological conditions such as rheumatoid arthritis, crystal arthropathies, or osteorathrosis. In some condition, such as adhesive capsulitis of the shculder, the restricted movements are due to capsular contracture. If the passive movements are restricted in a non-capsular pattern the possibility of intra-articular derangement arises; otherwise the periarticular structures are at fault.

Osteoarthrosis. Degenerative joint disease should be included in the differential diagnosis when the capsular pattern exists from the fourth decade onwards. The hips and knees are predominantly affected following years of competition in contact sports such as soccer. Although less common. AA of the upper limb joints may be secondary to previous fracture, or due to repeated joint-loading—for instance, from weight-lifting.

Synovitis. A synovial reaction may be secondary to

injury such as a ligament tear or a meniscus tear when it is associated with a serious effusion. Alternatively a serous effusion, accompanied by synovial tickening, amy be due to a rheumatological condition. Synovial irritation per se gives rise to the capsular pattern of restriction of movement. However, if synovitis is secondary to a mechanical derangement, such as a prolapsed meniscus or an intra-articular loose body, the signs resulting from the locked joint will prevail.

Hypomobility

The majority of acute traumatic incidents of all types give rise to local restriction of movement of the nearest joint: differentiation into articular and periarticular lesions is made by examination routine already described. The joint play movements—that is, movements that are not under control of the voluntary muscles—perform a particularly useful role in the diagnosis ad rehabilitation of spinal dysfunction. Peripheral joint dysfunction—that which is secondary to trauma or immobilization, for instance—also gives rise to loss of joint play.

Hypermobility

Although several terms are used in an interchangeable fashion, it is conventional to accept the following:

flexibility refers to a joint's range of motion—that is, it is principally a function of muscle/tendon tightness;

laxity refers to joint distraction and hear—that is, it is a function of ligamentous competence;

hypermobility refers to generalized joint laxity.

Hypermobility may be associated with connective tissue disorders such as Ehlers-Danlos and Marfan's syndromes. Even with no connective tissue disorder it is clear that some individuals have an inherited joint laxity. Although, at first sight, this would appear to be beneficial in, for example, gymnastics and dance disciplines such as classical ballet, there is an increased incidence of injury and osteoarthrosis in later life. Increased flexibility, resulting from training, may be best demonstrated by the ability to flex the spine and place the palms of the hands on the floor. Other hypermobile joints would not appear to be due to training, and only result from genetic disposition or in some cases injury.

The Beighton and Horan modification of the carter and Wilkinson index is often used:

(a) Passive apposition of thumbs to flexor aspects of the forearm—2 points.

(b) Forward flexion of the trunk with knees extended so that the palms rest flat on the floor immediately in front of the toes—1 points.

(c) Hyperextension of knees beyond 10°—2 points.

(d) Passive dorsiflexion of the little finger beyond 90°—2 points.

(e) Hyperextension of elbows beyond 10°—2 points.

Bursa

Bursae are synovial lined sacs whose function is to reduce friction between tendon and bone, or between skin and bone. Direct, particularly repetitive, trauma may give rise to inflammation in the more superficial bursae—for example, olecranon bursitis, prepatellar bursitis, and postcalcaneal bursitis. Alternatively, overuse of the overlying tendon may result in a chronic bursitis due to excessive friction—for example, trochanteric bursitis and iliotibial tract syndrome. In some situations the aetiology of bursitis may be multifactorial—for instance, the effects of rotator cuff degeneration and attrition under the coracoacromial arch on the development of subacromial bursitis. Burse are also a common site of soft tissue inflammation in such rheumatological conditions as gout or Reiter's syndrome.

Nerve

Nerve entrapment may result from overuse. Both the sensory and motor components of the larger-diameter myelinated fibres in peripheral nerves may be damaged by compression. A potentially reversible neuropraxia is the type of neuropathy found in the carpal tunnel and tarsal tunnel syndromes, in which entrapment occurs beneath an inflexible retinaculum. In other situations, such as compression of the radial or median nerves in the proximal forearm of weight-lifters and rowers, entrapment results from muscular hypertrophy. Alternatively, direct pressure may be responsible for such conditions as 'handlebar palsy' and acute compartment syndromes in the lower leg, affecting either the deep or superficial peroneal nerves. Spinal nerve roots may suffer entrapment due to HNP, from spinal canal stenosis or from an inflammatory reaction within the spinal canal that is secondary to trauma or overuse.

Muscle

The musculotendinous unit comprises a contractile element and a non-contractile element. Muscle fibres contain hundreds of thousands of myofibrils, each composed of approximately 1500 myosin filaments d twice that number of actin filaments. The myofibrils lie in parallel, and are responsible for te striated appearance of muscle; contraction results from these filaments gliding past each other.

Muscle fibres are not homogenous, several fibre types

have been identified using histochemical and physiological techniques. Red type I fibres are well endowed with mitochondria, and thus with oxidative enzymes; they fatigue slowly, and are found in muscles with predominantly fatigue slowly, and are found in muscles with predominantly antigravity or postural function, such as te soleus muscle. White type II fibres are principally anaerobic, using creatine phosphate and anaerobic glycolysis for release of energy; they fatigue quickly, and are fond in muscles requiring fast propulsive activity, such as the hamstrings and gastrocnemius muscles. Further analysis reveals that some type II fibres have relatively high potentials for oxidative metabolism, and there are leafed type IIA; others have a relatively low content of oxidative enzymes, and are called type II-B.

In addition to being a contractile unit, muscle acts as a shock-absorbing system; this is perhaps best illustrated by the automatic flexing of the knees that absorbs the shock through the legs when landing from a jump. Loss of shock-absorbing capacity predisposes to injury.

'Warm down' and post-exercise stretching prevent over-rapid cooling. Removal of lactic acid is best achieved at 40-60 percent of the previous level of activity.

Muscle may be injured by direct contusion, or by overload when excessive tension is applied to a contracting music. At a microscope level the initial biomechanical failure may occur in the interstitial music collagen lattice, although this view is conjectural. Fibre disruption occurs, with associated bleeding. Torn ends contract, and the defect fills with blood, subsequently becoming a clot invaded by fibroblasts and macrophages. If a complete tear occurs, dysfunction rather than pain is the predominant feature, and bleeding extravasates into the surrounding tissues. Partial tears may create a greater problem, as the developing haematom may be 'intramuscular' instead of 'extramuscular'. An intramuscular haematoma is more painful, and results in more prolonged rehabilitation. Occasionally it becomes cystic and requires surgical drainage.

During organization the intramuscular hematoma is gradually replaced by scar tissue. Although scar tissue remains inelastic, it may contract somewhat and become surrounded by hypertrophied muscle fibres, thus reducing the residual functional disability.

One complication of a severe contusion by direct trauma is the development of myositis ossifications. Ectopic ossification may manifest itself radiologically within ten days, the most common site being the quadriceps femoris, though it does occur elsewhere whenever muscle is deep and adjacent to underlying bone. Numerous theories have been proposed for the development of bone within music haematoma, including the migration of cells through damaged periosteum and crystalline calcification in necrotic tissue, leading subsequently to ossification. Whatever the cause, it appears to be a reaction by 'irritable muscle' to trauma, subsequently requiring a period of several months' rest to allow the bone to mature and contract. Of greater importance is the recognition of the risk of myositis ossificans, so that appropriate measures may be taken to prevent its onset.

Clinical assessment of muscle function involves four of the examination procedures previously described.

(a) Passive stretching, invoked by passive movement of the joint over which the muscle acts.

(b) Palpation—specifically for tenderness, the

presence of a defect, or a swelling.

(c) Observation of wasting.

(d) Resisted contraction, thereby imparting information on muscle strength and additionally on torn fibres. Strength may be graded 0-5 on manual testing.

Following an acute incident the patient's subjective awareness of pain on movement, and the resulting relative disability, are usually effective in stimulating early rest. Reduction of bleeding and stimulation of the repair phase are mainstays of treatment. However, there is often inadequate realization of the importance during rehabilitation of the two Ss: stretching the inelastic scar formation, and strengthening the weekend muscle unit. The main reason that muscle injuries such as hamstring tears have such a bad reputation for recurrence is that training is resumed before 100 % elasticity and 90 % of muscle strength have been regained.

Aetiological Factors in Oversue Injury

Oversue aetiological factors must be determined, and can be categorized as follows.

(I) Training surfaces, for example tarmac, tarta, flooring, canted, uneven.

(II) Growth factors i Children, such as size by size rather than age by age matching in contact sports, bone-muscle length ratios.

(III) Inadequate training schedules:

(a) intensity:

(b) frequency:

(c) overall loading:

(d) associated physiological fitness characteristics.

(IV) Equipment, for instance the suitability of footwear

or protective devices.

(V) Biomechanics:

(a) technique;

(b) joint mobility;

(c) musculotendinous balance and adequacy;

(d) inequality of limb length;

(e) malalignment.

Examples are legion, and will be described in the subsequent studies. Liaison with parent, coach, or trainer is often necessary. Repeated reassessment may reveal clues not evident on the patient's first visit. Other evidence—derived, for example, from video recording or treadmill running—may be required. Examination of footwear or equipment, as well as the patient, is advisable. Examination of those parts of the musculoskeletal system some distance away from the injured site is mandatory; an obvious example in distance running, for instance, is the study of foot biomechanics when faced with a presentation of low back or limb pain. Finally it must be remembered that slowly progressive pain may indicate a more serious pathology. From time to time osteoid osteoma presents in a similar fashion to a stress fracture; metastatic deposits may present as restriction of joint movement.

3

BASIS OF SPORTS INJURIES

Design and Fabrication

(i) Principles used to design protective pads

(a) Mechanical structuring-forces are reduced through the use of a mechanical structure

(b) Channelling-forces are channelled away from anatomical structures

(c) Restriction—range of motion is to prevent forces that cause injury

(iv) Dispersion-forces are dispersed over a larger area

(ii) Sound bio-mechanical and anatomical principles should be well thought out before a fabricated pad is placed on an athlete

Head and Facial Area

Helmets

Types

(i) Single or double air bladder

(ii) Closed-cell padding with air bladder

Selection

(i) Helmets can :

(a) Prevent skull fracture and conclusions

(b) Protect facial bones, eyes, nose, mouth, and ears

(ii) Mandatory for football, ice hockey, mens' lacrosse, baseball, soft-ball, bicycling, amateur boxing, and white water sports

Fitting

(i) Hair should be the length that the athlete will wear it for the season. If a haircut is done during the season, the helmet should be re-checked for proper fit.

(ii) Circumference of skull should be measured above the ears

(a) Most football helmet manufacturers will supply tape measure at no cost

(b) Manufacturer's taped measures will have suggested helmet size on reverse of tape

(iii) Proper sized shell is selected and front and back sizes and jaw pads are adjusted for a proper fit

(iv) Athlete should then:

(a) Put on helmet by tilting it backward and rotating it to the front while pulling it into position

(b) Spread the earflaps by placing the thumbs or fingers directly in the ear holes

(v) Helmet should be snug and Dover base of skull but not impinge the cervical spine when the neck is extended

(vi) Four-point chin strap should be used and be of equal tension and length on both sides

(vii) Proper fit in other helmets is achieved when a snug-fitting helmet does not move in one direction when the head is turned in the other

(viii) Riddell and AHI provide free educational materials on the care and fitting of helmets

(ix) Crown adjustment

(a) Press straight down on top of helmet

(b) Helmet should be 1-to-2-finger widths above the eyebrows

(c) Helmet should not move over the eyes

(x) Side to side

(a) Grasp the face mask pulling left then right; the helmet should not slip

(b) Jaw pads should not have any gaps between them and the face

(c) Ask athlete to look straight ahead and "pull" the helmet should not slip

(xi) Up and down

(a) Athlete should scalp hands behind the helmet and press forward

(b) Athlete should "bull" the neck and tug up and down on the face mask; the helmet should not slip

(c) Fitter should not be ale to place a finger

(xii) Each helmet should have:

(a) Detailed records that identify purchase date, use, reconditioning history, and certifications seals

(b) NOCSAE seal of approval adhered to the posterior right side of the helmet

(c) Date and tracking number engraved on the inside

(xiii) Each athlete should:

(a) Sign and date a statement that confirms he or she read the seal and have been informed of the risks of injury by improperly using the helmet or face mask when striking an opponent

(b) Statements should be signed, dated, and kept as part of the athlete's medical files

(c) Be given instructions in the proper use, fit, and care of the helmet

(d) Participate in a pre-season in-service program on safety

(e) Should read the NOCSAE seal

Selection and Fitting

(i) Major testing agencies include:

(a) Canadian Standards Association

(b) National Operating Committee on Standards for Athletic Equipment

(c) Sports Equipment and Facilities Committee of the American Society for Testing Materials

(ii) Those responsible for purchasing, fitting, and maintaining equipment must know certification standards for protective gear

(iii) Rules regarding legal equipment are established by:

(a) National Federation of State High School Association for interscholastic competition

(b) National sports governing bodies for international competition

(c) National Collegiate Athletic Association for intercollegiate competition

(iv) Football, baseball, and lacrosse helmets must have the NOESEA seal of approval permanently stamped ono rear of helmet; ice hockey helmets must have the CSA seal of approval; other helmets must meet ASTM standards

(v) When fitting protective equipment consider:

(a) Mandatory rules so proper insurance coverage is not compromised

(b) Body size, age, strength, physical development, and skill level of athlete

(c) Sport and position

(vi) Regardless of playing position or level of competition, all equipment issued must pass inspection in a court of law

Maintenance

(i) Inspect and recondition the equipment by professional reconditioners after each season

(ii) Check equipment on a weekly basis, and if damaged, replace immediately

(iii) Establish a master plan for purchasing, replacing, reconditioning, maintaining and tracking the equipment's use and age

(iv) Reconditioning/warranty standards for football helmet:

(a) ABS plastic shell helmets have a 2-year warranty

(b) AHI helmets should not be used more than 6 years

(c) All helmets should be reconditioned every-2 years

(d) Polycarbonate alloy shell helmets have a 5 years warranty

(e) Riddell helmets should not be used more than 10 years

Mouthguards

Selection

(i) Are mandatory and should

(a) Provide support to toothless space so partial dentures can be removed when appropriate

(b) Protect lips, cheek tissues, and gums

(c) number and severity of jaw fractures

(d) incidence of contusions

(e) risk of broken and chipped teeth, root and bone fractures

(ii) Mouthguards should:

(a) Cover all upper teeth except the last two molars

(b) Not hamper breathing

(c) Be durable, resilient, tasteless, odourless, resistant to tear, easy to fabricate

(d) Be visible to officials

(e) Stay in place when mouth is opened

Types

(i) Boxer-type guards made moulded rubber

(ii) Custom-fitted

(iii) Mouth formed—boil and dip

Fitting

(i) Place mouth-guard over upper dental arch

(ii) Rinse guard in cold a water to harden material

(iii) Immerse guard in boiling water for 20 to 30 seconds

(iv) Shake off excess water, but do not rinse in cold water

(v) Close mouth, but do not bring teeth together or bite down on guard

(vi) Suck as hard as possible for 15 to 25 seconds to mould guard around teeth

(vii) Check guard for imperfections on the bottom, and if present, select new guard and repeat the process

Face Guards

Types

(i) Heavy-gauge, plastic coated steel rod

(ii) Clear plastic

Selection

(i) No face mask should have less than 2 bars

(ii) Face guards must meet NOCSAE standards for strength and deflection

(iii) Eye shields can be attached

(iv) Depends on position played and desired protection

(a) Quarterbacks, running backs, and wide receivers wear an intermediate style for an unobstructed view

(b) Lineman wear full cage with middle bar to prevent

eye, nose, and facial injuries from opposing players' fingers

The Lower Body

Pelvis, Hip, and Thigh

Selection

(i) Depends on sport

(ii) Presence of pre-exiting injury

Types

(i) Girdle type pad is most effective for football, ice hockey, field hockey, and lacrosse goalkeepers

(ii) Thigh and hips pads

(a) Hard polythene covered with layers of Ensolite

(b) Neoprene

(c) Air management pads

(iii) Male genital region is best protected by a protective up in the athletic supporter

Fitting

(i) Girdle with pockets can hold hip, thigh, coccyx and genital pads in place

(ii) Thigh pads

(a) Should be centred over the quadriceps muscle group

(b) Asymmetrical thigh pads should have flared edge placed on lateral aspect of the thigh

(c) Should be placed 6 to 7 inches above the patella

Knee Braces

Selection

(i) Depends on:

(a) Physician recommendations

(b) Research and fit

(c) Proper diagnosis of condition

(ii) Functional knee braces provide stability for:

(a) Tedonitis

(b) Patellofemoral inflammations

(c) Ligament instability

(d) Bio-mechanical inefficiencies

(iii) Rehabilitation braces limit and protect knee ROM post-operative and non-post-operative

(iv) Prophylactic braces are worn to prevent or reduce incidence of knee injury

Type

(i) Functional

(ii) Prophylactic

(iii) Rehabilitative

Fitting

(i) Braces range from custom fitted braces to off-the-shelf models

(ii) Should be fitted according to manufacturer's

Lower Leg Protection

Selection

(i) Depends on:

(a) Proper diagnosis of condition

(b) Physician recommendations

(c) Rescarch and fit

(ii) Heel cups are used to reduce shearing and shock in the calcaneal region

(iii) Footwear selection is based on:

(a) Position

(b) Sport

(c) Playing surface

(d) Weather conditions

(e) Postural or mechanical problems

(iv) Shin guards should have high density pad covered by a moulded hard shell

(v) Commercial ankle supports:

(a) Comfort and support, will determine personal preference

(b) Should be used when ROM must be limited

(vi) Inner-soles made of Poron

(a) Provide a porous structure to absorb and disperse shock

(b) Can be used for an arthritic or diabetic foot

(vii) Semirigid orthotics

(a) Often used for fallen arches, pronated feet, or medial tibial stress-syndrome

(b) Provides a more stable and durable support for intrinsic foot structures

(viii) Rigid orthotics more effectively correct bio-mechanical malignant

(ix) Anti-shock heel lifts

(a) Use dense silicone mixture to cushion heel impact

(b) Can correct some bio-mechanical alignment

(c) Can relive strain on the Achilles tendon

Types

(i) Shin guards

(a) Hard, deflective plastic outer player with an inner layer of thin foam

(b) Plastic stays sewn into a felt material

(c) Hard, deflective plastic outer layer with an inner layer of thin foam

(ii) Inner-soles

(iii) Semirigid orthotics

(iv) Rigid orthotics

(v) Anti-shock heel lifts and cups

(vi) Footwear

(vii) Commercial ankle supports

(a) Lace-up brace

(b) Semirigid arthrosis

(c) Air bladder brace

Fitting

(i) Shin guards should extend from the tibial tuberosity and cover malleoli

(ii) Ankle supports and other protective equipment should be flitted according to manufacturer's guidelines

(iii) Footwear

(a) Shop at stores that employ professional sales people that work with the sport

(b) Athletes with a history of back, knee, ankle, or foot injuries may opt for a shorter multi-cleated design for stability and torsion forces

(c) Fit shoes at the end of the day or after practice

(d) Wear socks that would normally be worn during competition

(e) Fit shoe to longest lose

(f) Fit shoe to widest part of foot, usually forefoot

The Neck and Upper Body

Shoulder Pads

Types

(i) Flat type:

(a) Used when a great deal of mobility is needed

(b) Is light and allows full ROM at glenohumeral Joint

(ii) Cantilevered:

(a) Is often worn by running backs, linebackers and

defensive linemen

(b) is bulkier and has a device disperses impact forces over wider area of the body

Fitting

(i) Ice hockey and lacrosse pads:

(a) Pads are also sized for fit by measuring from AC joint to AC joint

(b) Pads must protect AC joint, clavicles, sternum, and shoulder cap

(ii) Sternum pads, rib protectors, and deltoid pads can supplement shoulder pads for extra protection

(iii) Football shoulder pads:

(a) Pads must be inspected weekly for cracks, loose or lose screws, or broke nor torn pads

(b) Measure across upper back from AC joint to AC joint

(c) Companies provide sizing charts to assist in selecting correct size for athlete

(d) Tip of the inside shoulder and should extend over lateral aspect of shoulder

(e) Pads should cover both scapulae, the sternum, clavicles, and extend 2 inches below nipple line

(f) Axillary and chest straps should be snug

(g) Neck opening should not impinge soft tissues of neck or slip when arms are abducted

Shoulder Harnesses

Selection

(i) Based on side specific

(ii) May be interchangeable on either shoulder

(a) Sully Brace can restrict excessive motion

(b) Prevents AC separations, and anterior or posterior dislocations

Types

(i) Several varieties available can restrict excessive abduction and external rotation

Neck rolls and Collars

Selection

(i) Depends on position played

(ii) May protect players with history of receptive burn or stingers

Types

(i) Wedge pad

(ii) External collar bolted to the pads

(iii) Round collar

(iv) Cowboy collar

Fitting

rolls and collars should never place the athletes neck in a flexed position

(a) Place cervical vertebrae in a fixed segmented column

(b) Risk of facial loading, which may result in catastrophic head or neck injury.

(ii) Fit to prevent hyperextension and lateral flexion of cervical vertebrae

Elbow, Forearm, Wrist, and Hand Protection

Selection

(i) Depends on condition and severity of injury

(ii) Material selection may be limited by sport governing bodies

Types

(i) Elbow braces

(a) Neoprene

(b) counter-force

(c) Hinge

(ii) Wrist and hand protection

(a) When immobilization is needed for fractures or sever sprains

(i) Silicone and fibreglass in preferred over heavier material

(ii) Can be worn during competition in must sports if padded properly

(b) Materials may include orthoplast, aquaplast, and plastazote

Environmental Considerations

Predisposing Factors to Heat Illness

(i) Children up to 12 years of age because they:

(a) Gain heat rapidly from the environment

(b) Lack judgement to understand impending symptoms of heat illness

(c) Sweat less efficiently

(d) Scclimate more slowly

(ii) Adults 55 or older because they:

(a) Have thirst mechanism when they become dehydrated

(b) Have less body water due to a lean body mass

(iii) Wheels chair athletes who do not like to drink fluids because of the inconvenience of urination

(iv) Diabetes that is uncontrolled

(v) Drugs: alcohol, amphetamines, cocaine, hallucinogens, laxatives, or narcotics

(vi) Poor acclimatization, poor physical condition, or obesity

(vii) Athletes with excessive muscle mass

(viii) History of heat illness

(ix) Medications: anticholinergics, diuretics, antihistamines, anti-beta—blockers, laxatives

(x) Heart disease or hypertension

(xi) Eating disorders

(xii) Electrolyte loss or dehydrated

Preventative Measures

(i) Weight records

(ii) Change practice time to a cooler time of the day

(iii) Cooling spray aperitive/competition

(iv) Gradual acclimatization

(v) Frequent fluid replacement readings

(vi) Temperature/humidity readings

(vii) Identify individuals with predisposing factors

(viii) Modify uniforms by wearing shorts, cut-off jerseys, no helmets, etc.

Causes

(i) Inadequate replacement of fluids

(ii) Evaporation of perspiration is blocked due to

(a) High humidity

(b) Protective equipment

(iii) Life-threatening medial emergency

(iv) All mechanisms for body cooling fail during later stages

Heat Stroke

Signs and Symptoms

(a) Gait is unsteady

(b) Disorientation and irritability

(c) Profuse seating

(ii) Late stages

(a) Pulse is rapid and strong

(b) Breathing is shallow

(c) Blood pressure

(d) Core temperature to 106°F

(e) Unconsciousness

(f) Seizes

(iii) As condition deteriorates

(a) Glassy stare, pupils dilated

(b) Skin becomes hot, dry, and red

(c) Sweating ceases

Organization Facilies

(i) Call EMS

(ii) Rapid cooling of the body

(a) Remote equipment and clothing

(b) Sponge the body with cold water or ice the major blood vessels in the axilla, groin, and neck

(c) Place athlete in a cold place

(d) Monitor vital signs until EMS arrives

(e) Use of fan, if available, or fan the athlete with a towel

(iii) Transport to a hospital as quickly as possible, continuing to cool the athlete during transport

Heat Exhaustion

Signs and Symptoms

(i) Skin calories ashen and gray

(ii) Skin is wet, col, and clammy

(iii) Core temperature; usually will not exceed 103°F

(iv) Pulse is rapid and weak

(v) Dizziness, lethargic, headache, fainting

(vi) Nausea

(vii) Uncoordinated gait

(viii) Blood pressure is low even in an upright position

(ix) Respiration is rapid and shallow

Organization Facilities

(i) If conscious, have athlete ingest cold clear fluids

(ii) Place athlete in a cool area

(iii) Remove all equipment and unnecessary clothing

(iv) Cool athlete by spongin or towelling him or her with cool water, particularly in the axilla, groin, and neck areas

(v) Take core temperature every 8 to 10 minutes making sure it does not exceed 106°F

(vi) Call emergency medical service

(vii) Monitor vital signs until EMS arrives

Heat Cramps

(i) Causea by imbalance between water and electrolytes in body from perspiration

Signs and Symptoms

(i) Involuntary muscle spasms

(ii) Fatigue

(iii) Nausea, vomiting

(iv) Headache

(v) Body Skin remains moist and cool

(vi) Pulse and respiration are normal or slightly elcvated

(vii) Skin remains moist and cool

Organization Facilities

(i) Rehydrate by drinking cool water

(ii) Ice the muscle on stretch

(iii) Athlete will generally not be able to return to participation that day

High-Altitude Pulmonary Edema

Cause

(i) Caused by lungs accumulating a small amount of fluids within the alveolar walls, which lead to pulmonary edema

Predisposing Factors

(i) Athlete of not acclimated to altitude

(ii) Athletes who are not native to or reside in the area

Signs and Symptoms

(i) Develops after symptoms of acute mountain sickness subside

(ii) Unconsciousness may occur

(iii) Fatigue and muscle weakness

(iv) Shortness of breath

(v) Headache and chest pain

(vi) respiration

(vii) Irritating cough with bloody, forth spectrum

(viii) Fatigue and muscle weakness

Organization Facilities

(i) Give oxygen, if available

(ii) Return to lower altitude immediately

(iii) Condition resolves quickly at lower altitude

Frostnip

(i) Often identified first by those around you

(ii) Affects the tips of ears, nose, cheeks, chin, fingers and toes

Signs and symptoms

(i) Slow, painless onset

(ii) No permanent tissue damage

(iii) Sudden blanching or whiteness of the skin

(iv) Slow, painless onset

(v) As warmth and colour returns, tingling may occur

(vi) Skin may turn red as warming occurs

(vii) Areas affected may peel or blister within 24 hours

Organization Facilities

(i) Apply firm steady pressure with a warm hand

(ii) Blow warm breath on the area

(iii) Do not rub the Area

(iv) Hold the nipped fingertips motionless in the axilla

Deep Frostbite

(i) A medical emergency

(ii) Usually affects hands feet but can affect ears, nose, cheeks, and chin

Organization Facilities

(i) Skin may permanently remain red, tender, and sensitive to re-exposure to cold

(ii) Transport athlete to the hospital/medical ability develop within 2 to 3 weeks

(iii) Take person indoors and do RAPID re-warning

(iv) Remove all jewellery and rings from fingers

(v) Immerse body part in warm water in a but large enough so the body part does not touch the sides or bottom

(vi) Pain and burning sensation may last for several weeks

(vii) If conscious, have athlete drinks hot clear fluids

(viii) Dry area after thawing, cover each digit individually with sterile gauze, and then over the entire area with towels or a blanket

(ix) In severe cases blisters will form and gangrene may develop within 2 to 3 weeks

Signs and Symptoms

(i) Skin appears cold, solid, and numb

(ii) As re-warming occurs:

(a) Extremely painful after thawing

(b) Swelling caused by capillary damage and plasma leaking into the tissue

(c) Skin will turn purplish blue

(iii) Firm, hard mass upon palpation with underlying tissues being rigid

Superficial Frostbite

(i) Affects the skin and underlying superficial tissue of the ears, nose, cheeks, chin, fingertips, and toes

(ii) Often identified first by individuals around you

Treatment

(i) A medical emergency

(ii) Usually affects hands and feet but can affect ears, nose, cheeks, and chin

Signs and Symptoms

(i) Skin appears pale, hard, cold, and waxy

(ii) Firmness upon palpation with underlying deeper tissues soft and resilient

(iii) As re-warming occurs:

(a) Swelling caused by capillary damage and plasma leaking into the tissues

(b) Skin may permanently remain red and sensitive to re-exposure to cold

(c) Athlete will first feel numbness, then stinging and burning sensations

(d) Skin will turn mottled blue or purple

(e) blisters may form

Predisposing Factors to Cold Injuries

(i) Fatigue or weakness

(ii) Inadequate protection from the cold or wind

(iii) Use of alcohol and other substances

(iv) Persons with Raynaud's phenomenon

(v) Inadequate diet and fluid intake

(vi) Restricted circulation from arterial disease or tight clothing, especially foot wear

(vii) Children:

(a) With asthma are prone to bronchoconstriction when breathing cold air

(b) Lose body heat faster than adults

(c) Are more prone to frostbite because of their enhanced peripheral vasoconstriction

(viii) Older adults are less able to adapt to cold from:

(a) Ability to vasconstrict peripheral arterials

(b) Rise in heat production during cold stress

Preventative

(i) Gradual acclimatisation

(ii) Replace fluids to avoid dehydration

(iii) Longer warm-up period during cold weather, or warm-up indoors when possible

(iv) Protect the body from heat loss within:

(a) Outer jacket

(b) Face mask and neck warmer

(c) Cap or hat

(d) Gloves

Causes

(i) Prolonged exposure to wet-cold conditions

(ii) Shivering through involuntary muscle contractions to generate heat ceases

(iii) Body heat loss exceeds body heat production

(iv) Vasoconstriction surface blood vessels prevent blood rom shunting to the skin

(v) heart, liver, brain, and endocrine organs

Altitude-Related Conditions Acute Mountain Sickness

Causes

(i) Caused by hypoxia at altitudes of 7000 to 8000 feet

Predisposing Factors

(i) Diet low in carbohydrates and high in sodium

(ii) Athletes who are not native to or reside in the area

(iii) Athlete not acclimated to altitude

Organization Facilities

(i) Return to lower altitude immediately

(ii) Give oxygen, if available

(iii) Condition resolves quickly at lower altitude

Signs and Symptoms

(i) Headache and dizziness

(ii) Insomnia

(iii) Nausea, vomiting

(iv) Fatigue

(v) Appetite suppressed

(vi) Tachycardia on exercises

(vii) Dyspnoea

Emergency Care

Unconscious Athlete

Causes

(i) Concussion

(ii) Respiratory distress

(iii) Metabolic disturbance

(iv) Syncope

(v) Drug overdose

(vi) Liver/kidney failure

(vii) Haemorrhage/shock

(viii) Cerebrovascular of cardiovascular malfunctions

(ix) Poising

(x) Seizure/epilepsy

(xi) Edema/infection affecting the brain-stem

Organization Facilities

(i) Determine level of consciousness through verbal and sensory stimuli

(a) Call the person's name

(b) Pinch soft tissue

(c) Tap your knuckles on his her sternum

(ii) Unless there are special circumstances, such as respiratory distress coupled with an inability to access the airway, the helmet should never be removed on the field when there is a potential head/neck injury

(iii) If individual does not respond

(a) Activate appropriate emergency medical system

(b) Immediately assess airway and circulation

(iv) Assume the presence of associate cervical spine trauma

(v) If airway is compromised and/or circulation is absent, stabilize the head and cervical spine and perform a log roll to position the athlete supine

(vi) Remove face mask if present. Note: if proper tools are not available CPR pocket mask can fit under face mask without having to remove it

(vii) If airway is intact and circulation is present, protect the athlete from further injury, perform a secondary survey, continue to monitor vital signs until emergency transport personnel arrive

CPR Emergencies

Causes

(i) Direct trauma

(ii) Electrical shock

(iii) Strenuous activity

(iv) Excessive alcohol or substance abuse

(v) Drowning

(vi) Suffocation

(vii) Heart anomalies

Organization

(i) Summon EMS

(ii) Follow standard first aid procedures for CPR .

Signs and Symptoms

(i) Pain originating behind the strum, which may radiate into one or both arms, the neck, jaw, teeth, upper back, or mid-abdomen

(ii) Feeling of impending doom

(iii) Nausea

(iv) Shortness of breath

Obstructed Airway

causes

(i) Solid foreign object

(ii) Swelling in the throat

(iii) Back of the tongue because of unconsciousness

(iv) Fluid

Organization Facilities

(i) Total airway obstruction

(a) Summon EMS

(b) Follow standard first aid procedures

(ii) Partial airway obstruction

(a) Reassure the individual you are there to help

(b) Allow individual to cough up object

Signs and Symptoms

(i) Partial airway obstruction

(a) Allows for some air exchange

(b) Individual exhibits choking behaviours

(ii) Complete airway obstruction

(a) Allows no air to pass

(b) Individual is unable to cough, speak, or breath

External Haemorrhage

Causes

(i) Requires removal from participation and prompt management to avoid infection and risk of disease transmission

(i) Shearing force coupled with tensile or compressive forces leading to exposed skin would

Organization Facilities

(i) Apply direct pressure with sterile gauze compressing the tissue firmly

(ii) Elevate the injured area about the heart

(iii) Put on latex gloves before you attempt to control haemorrhage

(iv) Apply indirect digital pressure to slow arterial bleeding

(v) Remove gloves, carefully turning them inside out to avoid contact with outer surface

(vi) Discard all blood-soaked gauze and gloves in a properly labelled biohazard container

Internal Haemorrhage

Causes

(i) Results from direct or indirect trauma

(ii) May occur in the presence of disease states leading to organ rupture

Organization Facilities

(i) Maintain an open airway

(ii) Continue to monitor vital signs until the ambulance arrives

(iii) Activate EMS

(iv) Monitor vital signs

(v) Check for fractures, splint if appropriate

(vi) Treat for shock

(vii) Loosen any restrictive equipment or padding at the neck and waist

(viii) Anticipate vomiting; place the individual on his or her side with the head downward, provided a spinal injury has been ruled out

(ix) Keep the individual calm and quiet

Signs and Symptoms

(i) Low blood pressure

(ii) Rapid, weak pulse

(iii) Bleeding from the mouth, rectum, or other body openings, bloody fluid from the nose or ears

(iv) Blood in the urine or urine output

(v) Nausea and vomiting blood

(vi) Severe respiratory distress; rapid breathing, possibly shallow

(vii) Pale, cold and clammy skin with profuse sweating

(viii) Feeling of impending doom, restlessness, or anxiety

(ix) Dull eyes, dilated pupils that are slow to respond to light

(x) pain, tenderness, swelling, or discoloration at the injury- site

Shock

Cause

(i) The inability of the heat to exert adequate pressure to circulate enough oxygenated blood to vital organs

(ii) Occurs as a result of:

(a) Vessel dilation leading to blood pooling away from vital areas

(b) Damaged heart

(c) Low blood volume from blood or dehydration

Predisposing Conditions

(i) Severe pain

(ii) Bleeding

(iii) Spinal injuries

Organization Facilities

(i) If you do not suspect a head or neck injury, or leg fracture, elevate the feet and legs 8 to 12 inches

(ii) If there are breathing difficulties, the individual may be more comfortable in a semi-recline position

(iii) With a head injury, elevate the head and shoulders to reduce pressure ono the brain

(iv) In a suspected neck and/or spine injury keep the individual lying flat

(v) If the individual vomits or is unconscious, place the athlete on his or her side to avoid blocking the airway with any fluids. This allows the fluids to drain from the mouth

(vi) Do no give the athlete anything by mouth

(vii) Monitor vital signs every 2 to 5 minutes until the ambulance arrives

(viii) Active EMs immediately

(a) Control any major bleeding and monitor vital signs

(b) Secure and maintain an open airway

(ix) Splint any fractures to reduce pain and limit shock

(a) Raise the leg only after it has been properly immobilized

(b) With a leg fracture, keep the leg level while splinting

(x) Move the individual to a warm environment

(a) Maintain body heat

(b) Remove any wet clothing if possible, and cover the individual with a blanket

Fractures and Dislocations

Causes

(i) Axial compression

(ii) Tensile forces that may or may not be combined; with shearing forces

Organization Facilities

Principles of Splinting

(i) Establish an open airway and complete the primary survey

(ii) Check the distal pulse and sensation

(a) if pulse is weak, check for internal haemorrhage

(b) If sensation is altered, summon EMS

(iii) Remove any clothing and jewellery around the injury site. Clothing should be cut away with scissors to avoid moving the injured area

(iv) Cover all wounds, including open fractures with sterile dressings and secure them

(v) Do not attempt to push the bone ends back underneath the skin

(vi) Pad the splint to prevent local pressure

(vii) Apply minimal in line traction and maintain it until splint is in place and secured

(viii) Air splints should not be used for an open fracture

(ix) Splint firmly, but do not impair circulation

(a) Re-check distal pulse and sensation after applying splint

(b) Check vital signs

(c) Arrange transport to a medical facility

(x) Immobilize the joint above and below the fracture site

(a) With such injuries, immobilize in the position you find the limb in, moving it as little as possible during splint application

(b) If pain with gentle traction or the limb resists positioning, splint in the position found

(c) Severely angulate fractures should not be straightened unless it is absolutely necessary to incorporate limb into splint

Types of Splints

(i) Rigid splints are commercially available and are:

(a) Made of wood, aluminium, wire, cardboard, or plastic

(b) Designed in specific shapes for upper and lower extremities

(ii) Choice of splint is determined by site of fracture and availability of splinting materials

(iii) Pneumatic splints are soft and pliable prior to inflation and:

(a) Become rigid once inflated

(b) Can have a radiograph through it

(iv) Vacuum splints

(a) Work by removing air from the splint, causing a rigid supportive structure

(b) Can have a radiograph though it

(v) Traction splints

(a) Provide counter pull to immobilize bone ends and prevent further injury

(b) Immobilize long bones

(vi) Improvised splints

(a) Be light yet rigid

(b) Can be made from a cardboard box, magazine, newspaper, or shin guard

(c) The surface next to the skin should be padded

(d) Should and below the injury

Epiphyseal Fractures

(i) Account for over 15% of all fractures to adolescents

(ii) Classified in Salter–Harris categories according to risk of disruption of blood supply and growth arrest

(a) Type I: complete separation of epiphysis, no fracture through bone

(b) Most II: most common, involves the plate and a triangular segment of the metaphysis

(c) Type III: plate injury extends through articular cartilage into the joint

(d) Type IV: fracture extends through articular cartilage into the joint, and into the metaphysis

(e) Type V: crushing injury to epiphyseal plate

Organization Facilities

(i) Type I and II: managed with immobilization and have a good prognosis if the blood supply is intact

(ii) Type III and IV: managed with immobilization and internal fixation, however, prognosis for Type IV is poor

(iii) V is managed with non—weight-bearing g for 3+ weeks to prevent compression also and has a poor prognosis

Spinal Cord/Neurologic Injuries

Causes

(i) May result in life-threatening and/or catastrophic injuries to the spine central nervous system

(ii) May occur secondary to head trauma

Signs and Symptoms

(i) Pain on palpation

(ii) Burning pain that radiates

(iii) Weakness in a myotome

(iv) Reduced or absent reflexes

(v) Complete paralysis

(vi) Numbness, tingling, or loss of sensation in a dermatome

(vii) Muscles spasm

Management

(i) Observe body position

(ii) Assess level of consciousness

(iii) Determine presence of head, neck, or back pain

(iv) Assured pupil size, reactivity, and movement

(v) Check eyes, nose, and ears for the presence of blood and/or fluid

(vi) Palate spine and skull

(vii) Functional assessment: memory, cognitive function, behaviour, balance, and coordination

(viii) Assess neurologic function: cranial nerves and spinal nerves

(ix) Unless there are special circumstances, such as respiratory distress coupled with an inability to access the airway, a helmet should never be removed on the field where there is a potential head/neck injury

(x) Immobilize on spine board with constant stabilization of the head, neck, and spine

(xi) When vital signs are compromised CPR must be initiated immediately after positioning the athlete on the spine board.

4

PRINCIPLES OF MANAGEMENT OF SPORTS INJURIES

Sports injuries can be broadly classified into two bıg groups overuse injuries and traumatic injuries. Traumatic injuries are fairly straight forward in their origin. Overuse injuries are a result of exercise induced micro-damage accumulating past the point where the body is able to repair, hence manifesting as clinical injuries. Another common cause of injury is too soon too fast. This usually happens when an athlete starts on a new exercise programme and experts unrealistic progress, advancing faster than the body's ability to cope resulting in injury.

A rule of thumb of increment would be about 10 per cent increase per week in your exercise regime. Some more gifted athelets may be able to advance faster than this but this is a safe margin for most. I like to draw an annalogy between progress in exercise and the snake and ladde board game. All of us like to make leaps and bounds in our exercise progress, not unlike the ladder in the boundgame, however, be ever mindful of the ugly snake waiting quietly at the corner, like an injury, which will undo your progress ad return you to square one.

What should be done when injuries occured?

The management of sports injuries can be approached from 1 angles, the acute on field management and definitive treatment. Acute on the field management includes moving the casualty to a safe place. ABCs of resuscitation if necessary and RICE therapy. RICE therapy is an acronym for Rest, Ice, Compression and Elevation. The injured body part must be allowed to rest to facilitate recovery.

The body intrinsic natural response to injury is pain and it is primarily protective. No pain no gain does not apply here! Ice is useful to encourage blood vessels to contract and therefore reduce the amount of bleeding and hence swelling. Swellings around the joint have been shown to be inhibitive to muscles contraction, another inbuilt protective reflex. Compression in the form of bandages is useful to limit a laurniquet! Finally elevate the injured part to facilitate circulation and minimize swelling.

Now, What's Next?

The first principle in the management of sports injuries is to get an accurate diagnosis. Simple as it may sound, it is often overlooked. How many of you are guilty of self medication without a proper diagnosis, only to seek attention later and realize it is not a muscle pull as you had thought. An accurate precise diagnosis, sometimes necessitating diagnostic aids such as ultrasound and MRI is the key foundation to the management of any sports injuries. It forms the roadmap to a formulation for recovery and treatment plans. So see your doctor and find out what's wrong first!

The next step is to relieve pain and swelling. This is an important step to contain the damage and to facilitate the body repair mechanisms. This may entail the use of medications, physiotherapy etc. Rehabilitative exercise may be initiated at this point to facilitate return of range of motion exercises. Treatment goals are clearly identified and a team approach is adopted. Sports medicine is one specially where a team comprising of coach, trainer, team physician, sports therapist and the sports orthopedic surgeon works together to draft cut a recovery plan for the patient.

Having diagnosed the problem, the next and probably the most difficult step is to identify the root cause. Sports injuries are notoriously difficult to eradicate because they keep recurring. The reason behind is that the athlete keeps infliciting the same injury on himself when he return to the sports after you have treated him. How? Well, the answer lies in understanding the biomechanics and nature of the game and the demand it places on the body.

All example would be the relationship between cricket bowlers and shoulder injuries. The bowler uses an overhead throw with a fairly straight arm, placing tremendous stress on the shoulder joint. A firm understanding of the bowler technique will help to pick up bowling technique errors which can help to prevent a recurrence besides just treating the shoulder injuries.

Although in the management of sports injuries, therapy and medications form the main pillar of treatment, in selected cases surgery may be required. One of the big advances in the surgical management of sports injuries have been the use of keyhole surgery. The advantage of keyhole surgery is the damage to unaffected tissues is extremely smaller, facilitating much faster recovery and return to sports. In addition, the results are just as good if not better than conventional open surgical techniques. Such techniques are widely applied to many parts of the body like the knee, shoulder, wrist, ankle and the spine.

Finally, the last tenet of sports injury management is a gradual and safe return to sports. Remember the snake and ladder board game! Realistic goals should be set and pace yourself. A common misconception is to pick up where you last left off, i.e. before you get injured 6 months ago. I would suggest dropping to at least 50% of where you left off and build up gradually.

In summary, accurate diagnosis with a team approach to the management of sports injuries will put many athletes on the road to recovery. Identification of root causes either in techniques or training programmes will minimize recurrences and finally a graduated but safe return to sorts.

SPORTS INJURIES AND MANAGEMENT

Sports injuries are injuries that occur most commonly during sports or exercise. They can be due to poor training, inadequate warm up, lack of conditioning, or trauma. Learn about various sports injuries and how the best ways to prevent and treat them.

Common Baseball Injuries

Baseball is a fun summer sport, but can also result in a few common injuries. Learn more about the injuries you are at risk for while playing this great past time.

Common Sports Injuries

Athletes often sustain injuries when performing sporting activities. Review the most common sports injuries

Achilles Tendonitis

An overview of Achilles tendonitis, including symptoms, prevention, and management.

Ankle Sprains

A review of the symptoms and management of ankle sprains, using physical therapy.

Icing an Injury

Icing an injury helps to slows the inflammation and

swelling that occurs after damage to a muscle, tendon, or ligament.

ACL Injuries

ACL injuries are among the most common sport related knee injuries. Approximately 100,000 – 200,000 people in the United States acquire a torn or ruptured ACL every year.

Runner's Knee

Jumpers knee, also known as patellar tendonitis, occurs when the patellar tendon becomes inflammed.

Patellofemoral Syndrome

Patellofemoral Syndrome is a condition where the patella does not track correctly on the femur. As a result, knee pain is experienced with activity.

Risk Factors for Stress Fractures

A review of the risk factors for stress fractures.

Common Running Injuries

Running makes people more susceptible to certain injuries of the legs. Review a few of the injuries in this article.

Shin Splints

Shin splints are an overuse injury that results in pain along the lower leg area. Learn more about shin splints in this profile.

Groin Strain

A groin strain results when the adductor muscles of the thigh are overstretched.

Ankle Sprain Treatment

The McKinley Health Center provides a comprehensive look at the management of an ankle sprain.

Golfer's Elbow

Golfer's elbow is an inflammatory disorder of the muscles that flex the wrist.

Iliotibial Band Syndrome

Iliotibial band syndrome is an inflammatory disorder that affects the lateral thigh and knee.

Runner's Knee

Runner's knee, or patellofemoral syndrome, is caused by the patella bone rubbing on the femur. Review the symptoms, causes, and management of runner's knee.

Stress Fractures

A stress fracture is an overuse injury that results when muscles are over worked. Read this article to learn more about stress fractures and how to treat them.

Turf Toe

Turf toe is a sprain at the base of the base toe. Learn what causes this injury and where its name came from.

Tennis Elbow

Tennis elbow is an injury not only experienced by tennis players. Learn the cause and symptoms.

The Unhappy Triad

The Unhappy Triad involves an injury to three specific structures of the knee. Learn what these structures are and how this injury occurs.

Sprain Vs. Strain

A review of the difference between strains and sprains.

Rest, Ice, Compression, Elevation - Management of Acute Injuries

RICE is an acronym used for the initial management

of acute sports injuries. Learn how to put these steps into effect.

Turf Toe

All you need to know about the causes, symptoms, and rehabilitation of turf toe are reviewed by MedFriendly.

Exercises to Rehab a Sprained Ankle

Use these rehabilitation exercises to regain strength in your sprained ankle and help prevent future injury.

Runner's Knee

Runner's knee is a commonly experienced disorder. Learn the medical name of this condition and how to treat it.

Tennis Elbow

Tennis elbow is caused by an inflammation of the tendons that extend the wrist. Review an in depth description of this disorder and multiple rehabilitation exercises in the management of tennis elbow.

Golfer's Elbow

Spent too much time on the golf course? Review the cause, symptoms, and management of golfer's elbow.

5

CARE AND PREVENTION OF SPORTS INJURIES

Liability of the Medical Profession in Sports Injury

Members of the medical profession, in particular those involved with sports injuries, have a responsibility to advise both sports groups and individuals on aspects of prevention of injury resulting from sport. Such advice may be offered at al levels, with the recipients ranging from sports governing bodies on the one hand to local sports clubs and individual sports participants on the other. Major strides in injury prevention have been made in certain directions, though progress is slow in others, particularly where there are financial implications and where there are possibilities of infringement of personal freedom. This advisory function should be the responsibility not on of the various association of sports physicians on behalf of their membership, but also of individual practitioners, acting in concert with administrators, managers, and coaches in their own localities.

Protective Equipment of Sports

Reduction in the incidence of injury due to direct trauma is influenced by the design of protective equipment and the obligation upon the wearer to comply with the regulations of sports associations. An obvious example is the wearing of suitable helmets by horse-riders. In horse-racing the wearing of a skull cap of acceptable design is mandatory. In competition under the control of the British Horse Society or the Pony Club it is also compulsory for the riders to wear a protective helmet that conforms to British Standards Institute regulations BS 4472 or BS 6473. However many competitions are not held under such control, with inevitable consequences. Even when a helmet is worn, it is important to stress the need for attachment of the chinstrap. Of course, flashion plays a part. Not long ago Mike Brearley was advocating the use of head and facial protection while batting at cricket. At first, the reaction from the 'macho' element was of disbelief, but the application of protection in specific risk situations, for example bating or fielding close to the wicket, is now commonplace. In some sports, such as American football, motorcycling, cricket, and hockey, the helmet has a visor or grille extension to reduce the incidence of maxillofacial injury. Standards and statutory requirements vary in different sports: in some it is also necessary to comply with international regulations.

In American football body protection has become so extensive that the sceptic is inclined to the view that he game is effectively a licence to injure. However, the incidence of head, neck, and shoulder injuries appears to be on the decline. In cricket batsmen often protect the forearms and thighs as well as the genitals. In karate the use of fit pads has been shown to reduce the severity of head injuries, which account for the majority of injuries sustained in tournaments.

Goggles are worn in a number of sports in which high speeds are encountered. Special goggles made from tough polycarbonate material are available for squash, though to date none are approved by the Squash Rackets Association. However, one should not assume that the mere replacement of spectacles by contact lenses protects the eye. Increased damage to the eye may result from direct trauma to a contact lens; soft lenses are safest.

Mouth guards are compulsory in some sorts, for example boxing, and their use is encourage though not mandatory in others, such as rugby football. All contact sports participants are at risk; the highest incidences of injury to the mouth and teeth are in rugby football in the UK and American football in the USA. 'Non-contact' sports participants are not exempt, as direct trauma in these sports is to uncommon. It has been mandatory for some time for all high school and college footballers in the USA to wear mouth protectors: in the UK progress has been somewhat slower. A suitable protector acts against trauma to the teeth, fittings, bridges, and crowns. Additionally, the likelihood of laceration of lips, mouth, and tongue from the teeth is drastically reduced, as are mandibular fractures and concussion injury which may result from the teeth being forcefully clenched together by an impact from below.

A number of different mouth guards are available. 'Off the shelf' guards are the least adequate, as they may fit badly and easily be displaced. An inexpensive guard made from a theromoplastic material, for instance a polyvinyl acetate-polyethylene polymer, and moulded by the patient usually fits better, though it may not be sufficiently extensive or resilient at point of maximal stress. A custom-made mouth guard constructed from a cast impression taken by a dental surgeon is the most satisfactory. A number of different materials are available; however, the cost is considerably higher than in te non-custom-made types.

The designs of ski boots has helped to reduce certain types of injury such as ankle fractures, though to some extent these have been replaced by boot-top tibial fractures. 'Modern two-mode ski-release bindings have allowed earlier release of the ski under excessive rotational stress, and thereby reduced the incidence of grade I medial collateral ligament knee injuries, though not the more severe knee ligament disruptions. Proper care of bindings help to reduce incidence of injury. It is also possible that further sophistication in the release system, for example from the present-day sensitivity to forward lean at the posterior attachment and twist at the toe, to a multimode system, might lower the incidence of lower-extremity injury still further.

Attention to specific clothing is important in certain sports for example, the use of fireproof material for racing drivers, and the utilization of neoprene, reinforced by nylon, in the manufacture of water-skiing pants to prevent vaginal or rectal douches. Light-weight emergency anti-exposure clothing should be carried by hill-walkers and mountain-climbers to protect against sudden changes in the weather.

Sports arenas

Safety designs of arenas and training and competition surfaces, including pole-valuating, high jump, and gymnastic landing areas, are important considerations. In gymnastics the basic basement requirement of 1½ inches of padding should be augmented by mats of 4 inch thickness around the various pieces of equipment. Suitable padding of essential props reduces the incidence of direct traumatic injury. Spring-back flag posts of non-breakable material should be used. Injuries to the thumb on dry-ski slopes may result from a fall in which the thumb is caught in the diamond-shaped gaps between the links. It seems likely that the incidence of this type of injury will be reduced when skiing on other recently introduced artificial surfaces. Indoor arenas should be designed to exclude obstacles such as radiators, which are potential sources of injury.

Pre-participation screening

Guidelines on individuals' fitness to complete should be established in co-operation with the relevant sports bodies. The practice of medical screening prior to participation in sport varies enormously from country to country. On the basis of prevention of illness and injury, screening makes sense. As an example, the existence of hyperextension of the knees or hypermobility in general should result in a ban from contact sports because of the risk of ligament and/or joint injury. In the UK, however, he provision of such screening services within the framework of a National Health Service that is already stretched in other directions is debatable. Nevertheless a healthy debate should include the advocacy of a changing emphasis in health care towards prophylaxis against injury.

Participation in certain sports or recreational activities such as subaqa diving requires a medical examination and certification of fitness. Other sports require medical certification if the participant has reached a certain age—for example, is over 40 in parachuting. It is of some interest that people with certain medical conditions are prevented from parachuting, whereas there is no proscribed level of lower-limb musculoskeletal incompetence. Participation in the majority of sports in the UK does not require any statutory examination procedure.

A suitable pre-participation medical examination which encompasses the techniques described in individually is summarized as follows:

Technical Factors in Overuse Injury

Reduction in incidence of overuse injury is dependent upon the prior identification of the relevant aetiological factors responsible for overload. Thus excessive or abnormal biomechanical stress, caused by poor sports technique or associated with anatomical malalignment, needs modification by appropriate means. Further stress reduction should be achieved by the choice of suitable sports shoes and equipment. Training schedules should be critically assessed in conjunction with coaches ad trainers—excessive training may improve some physiological parameters, but often leads to biomechanical injury.

Racket construction

Over the last few years artificial materials such as graphite and boron have been used increasingly in racket construction. Although unsubstantiated at present, it may be demonstrated later that the incidence of forearm and elbow overuse injury has been altered for the worse by this trend. Sports physicians should monitor the incidence of injury so as to be ale to advise on future construction patterns in the manufacture of sports equipment.

Sports shoes

There has been a consistent improvement in design of running shoes over the last decade. Excellent texts describing the construction of shoes are available, and a detailed account will not be reproduced here. However, one or two relevant general points should be made. An unsatisfactory level of support or shock absorption may be associated with the following:

(i) inadequate heel counter;

(ii) inadequate arch support

(iii) destruction between the upper and the sole;

(iv) an inadequate shoe, for example a casual 'trainer' or squash shoe, being chosen instead of a running trainer;

(v) distortion occurring in the worn shoe;

(vi) early deterioration of the sock-=absorbing properties of the midsole;

Pressure effects, giving rise to bursitis or tendinitis, may be due to the following:

(i) insufficient breadth of shoe;

(ii) biomechanical abnormalities;

(iii) laces that are too tight;

(iv) laces that are too tight;

(v) anatomical foot deformities;

The overall level of medial arch support is often inadequate. The flimsy insole that is so often provided in running shoe may be replaced by a more substantial commercially available arch support. An orthotic may be required for correction of excessive biomechanical stresses. Orotic appliances are used realign an abnormally balanced foot by controlling either the subtalar joint or the forefoot. A temporary 'soft' orthotic may be constructed in the surgery by the use of small pads of chiropody felt positioned on to a flexible insole: support under the medial arch and under the medial aspect of the heel is useful for overpronators. For greater sophistication, and for a long-term approach, a more rigid orthotic should be manufactured from a cast of the patient's foot made by an orthotist or podiatrist. The foot is cast in subtalar neutral; a positive mold is formed from this plaster cast by pouring in moulding plaster. Suitable posting may be added to correct deformities. The ortotic is the constructed using one of a number of materials, according to the ortotist's or the manufacturer's inclination.

The most common reason for the use of ortotics is correction of compensatory overpronation of the foot associated with conditions such as forefoot varus. Less satisfactory results are obtained with the supinated foot. Orthoses may be used to prevent injury or the recurrence of injury, or be part of the therapeutic armamentarium that is used for established conditions, such as metatarsalgia, plantar fascitis, 'runner's knee', and illiotibial tract bursitis, when there are identifiable biomechanical foot abnormalities.

In comparison with running shoes, which have thick soles to reduce impact, squash shoes provide greater stability , as they allow the foot to be closer to the ground.

Malalignment

Femoral anteversion in young dancers increases the likelihood of lower limb injury. Excessive internal rotation of the hips, detected most easily when a patient is examined in the prone position, is suggestive of femoral anteversion. The additional features of squinting patellae and excessive Q-angle are poor prognostic indicators for athletes contemplating long-distance running. Both pes cavus and pes planus are associated with increased incidence of foot and lower limb injury. Performance targets should be adjusted accordingly.

Flexibility

Lack of flexibility in one or more joints may be found during medical examination or noted by the trainer/ coach. It may be congenital—for example, the cavoid foot. Alternatively it may be due either to intrinsic joint pathology or to a lack of elasticity of the surrounding musculotendinous structures. Athletes generally may not receive appropriate advice on the relevance of stretching exercises, or may become non-compliant as a result of boredom, shortage of time, or for other reasons. It is of the utmost importance that exercise is preceded and followed by a flexibility programme for al major muscle groups to help prevent injury. Using dance as a example, considerable hip extension is required for arabesque; restriction of extension results in pelvic sway and excessive lumbar lordosis. Hamstring muscle tears and tendinitis are common if the hamstrings are to regularly stretched. Cyclists may also develop hamstring tendinitis, and therefore should utilize a stretching routine. Long-distance runners who have a 'shuffling' gait tend to develop limited hip movement as a result of soft tissue contracture, and are prone to pelvic stress injuries. Squash players are liable to back injury due to the combination of flexion and rotational stresses on he thoraco-lumbar spine; inadequate spinal flexibility compounds this risk. To help prevent subacromial problems in swimmers and tennis players and adequate warm-up should include a comprehensive stretching routine for the shoulders.

Technique

It is apparent that inadequate technique throws abnormal biomechanical strains upon the athlete's musculoskeletal system; examples are given throughout the text. Vigilance is required by the teachers and coaches in order to prevent injury from poor technique. The incidence of low back problems, including spondyloysis, in young dancers should be kept to a minimum by attention to posture in certain exercises. Thus are should be taken to avoid an excessive lordosis to the barred and in floor exercises dancer a correct lifting technique is necessary to reduce lordotic stress. The foundation of properdance technique is a strong well-balanced lumbar spine and pelvis. Excessive pelvic flexion or extension will undermine technique and increase the likelihood of injury.

The pivot area of the spine, the lumbosacral junction,

is also at particular risk in other sports if technique is faulty. Too much forward swing prior to powerful leg action in rowers should be corrected. Hyperflexion and hyperextension, both in the air and on water-entry, is a cause of low back injury in high board divers. Overuse of the butterfly stroke is a further cause of low back pain in swimmers. In weight-training, injury risk may be lessened by preventing spinal flexion on attempting heavier loads.

Technique is particularly important in the various field athletics disciplines. In javelin throwing, for instance, power is maximized by rotation of the chest and body. During the throw, the knee ipsilateral to the throwing arm is brought through quickly to block forward momentum and 'square off' the body, thereby reducing the likelihood of a side-arm throw, which is more likely to incur shoulder strain. Varying degrees of upper body rotation are utilized in the different throwing styles.

In other sports, such as Alpine skiing, it is clear that technical guidance from qualified instructors may reduce the incidence of certain types of injury—for example, reduction of likelihood of injury to the first MCP joint by excluding the thumb from the leather wrist strap.

Bicycle maintenance

Bicycles should be regularly overhauled, not only to prevent accidents resulting from major structural faults, but also to reduce the likelihood of the insidious onset of overuse injury due to abnormal biomechanical stress. In particular, emphasis should be given to he pedal-crank-bottom-bracket axle inter-connections. Excessive wear or poor adjustment may result in patellofemoral pain.

Biomechanics

A basic knowledge of sports mechanics is required to

appreciate the factors involved in prevention of injury, aetiology of injury, and management of injury. Consideration should be given to such concepts as force torque, centre of gravity, and lever arms. The axis of rotation itself has great relevance in certain joints such as the subtalar joint. In other joints the resultant force in different positions of the surrounding levers is of greater relevance—for example, in the patellofemoral joint. Of course, muscle function depends on its physiological state of training. Its force of contraction depends on cross-section, and its effectiveness on its position in relation to a point. The ground-reactive forces—that is, those forces which are applied to the body by contact with the ground—depend on the magnitude of the force with which the athlete presses on the ground. Such external vertical forces amount to two and ha half to three times the body-weight in running, and may increase to three or four times the bodyweight in jumping, and to even lighter levels on bouncing. Therefore, activities such as the more aggressive forms of 'aerobics' impose considerable repetitive strains on the legs, commonly resulting injuries such as Achilles tenditinitis and shin splints. The suitability of sock absorption, either in the training shoe or the training surface, is an important consideration in the prevention of these injuries.

The mechanics involved in locomotion in its various forms, and the technical requirements of various sports, may not be obvious in particular individual without more refined study. Video recordings that allow slow-motion playback of running style on a treadmill, EMG tests, stress plate analysis, high-speed motion photography, and discussions with the trainer or coach are all ways of identifying faults. Some of the instrumentation is available principally as a research tool, though increasing use is now made of video analysis in the clinical setting. The qualified coach or trainer is familiar with kinetics and dynamics, so that under his guidance suitable flexibility and strengthening regimes are included in the athlete's training programme. The sports physician should also develop a suitable baseline of knowledge of kinesiology and be able to relate this to clinical problems. For example, in sprinting, high knee action is coupled with early elevation of the heel towards the bullock as soon as the foot leaves the ground—rapid leg movement is achieved by the use of a small swing radius. Strong hip flexors and knee flexors are required. Training should concentrate on strengthening these muscles, and creating a balance with the gluteals and the quadriceps. Routine stretching of all these muscle groups is equally important, and in hurdlers is particularly necessary for the hamstrings.

The running style of long-distance runners is quite different; muscle economy is required. The running style is more of a shuffle, with little hip movement. Although powerful hamstrings are not required, nevertheless the athlete is at risk of developing hamstring contracture unless flexibility exercises are performed regularly. Poor elasticity of the hamstrings creates a risk of muscle 'pull' during bursts of activity—for example, in downhill running—that invoke greater stretch.

Further biomechanical considerations are identified by reference to the following examples, which are particularly relevant to a number of sports.

Quadriceps femoris exercises

The rectus femoris flexes the hip and extends the knee. The vastus lateralls and intermedius extend the knee only. The vastus medialis obliquus stabilizes the patella by pulling it medially. Examples of exercises which strengthen the knee extensor components of the quadriceps femoris are as follows:

(i) squat jumps;

(ii) 'sitting' against a wall with both hips and knees flexed to 90°;

(iii) step-ups, particularly when extra load is applied by carrying free weight;

The muscle force increase as knee flexion increases. Patellofemoral compression also increases alarmingly at the extreme of flexion—up to as much as eight times the bodyweight. Thus it may be seen that zero force is required to maintain the extended knee. i.e. in the upright position, and the VMO is not exercised significantly in these regimes.

Following injury, however, it is necessary to develop the VMO at the onset: are likelihood of patellofemoral in is high if isotonic exercises are performed too early. Thus therapists take patients through a carefully graded sequence of straight. Subsequently, progressive resistance training is performed using weights from flexion through to extension. Many gymnasts contain items of equipment which load the knee concentrically in this way. However, when this type of exercise is undertaken the patellofemoral joint is increasingly loaded, and the quadriceps work increasingly hard in extension, not flexion. This is an unnatural situation for most everyday activities and sports. When 'unnatural' stress is applied, for instance when the relatively untrained or the skeletally immature engage in unsupervised exercise using gymnasium equipment that utilizes a weight-stack resistance principle, particularly the leg-press station, the risk of injury is significantly raised.

Abdominal muscle exercise

Well-developed abdominal muscles are required to stabilize the spine, acting as antagonists to the paraspinal extensors. They also reduce shear strains by their action on the dorsilumbar fascia, and unload pressure on the intervertebral discs during lifting. The extensors are rarely weak, either in athletes or in the general pcpulation, as they are postural muscles. However, the abdominals are often relatively weak: abdominal strengthening exercises are thus useful for all. A critical study of exercises which are commonly prescribed for abdominal strengthening reveals a need for differentiation between abdominal muscle contraction and hip flexor contraction. When hanging from a bar and raising the legs to the horizontal, or lysing supine and raising both legs in the air, he iliopsoas contracts powerfully. There is a considerable transmission of force to the lumbar spine, increasing intradiscal pressure and increasing lordosis, thereby incurring risk of injury to the lumbar spine in those individuals who do not have established strong abdominal musculature. To off-load the spine and yet exercise the abdominals instead of te hip flexors, trunk curl exercises should be performed in a specific way. In the supine position the hips and knees are flexed as far as possible and the feet flexed to 90°. In this way the hip flexors are disengaged. Curled trunk sit-ups strengthen the rectus abdominal, and angulations to each side strengthen the external and internal obliques. Commonly, exercises are performed in less hip flexion with the ankles/feet supported under a wall bar for example. Although the lumbar lordosis has been abolished to a considerable degree in this position, the iliopsoas is able to assist the abdominals. The earlier part of the sit-up is by concentric abdominal contraction, and the latter half is by concentric iliopsoas contraction.

Although elitist athletes are ale to perform multiple hip flexor repetitions, the relatively less fit or those recovering from injury, particularly back strain, require expert guidance in the first instance on the correct way to exercise the abdominals in isolation.

Biomechanics of running

The terms 'overpronation', 'podiatric assessment', and provision of 'orthosis' have become familiar to many competitive athletes, who may assume that functional support in the running shoe is an important factor in prevention of injury. It behaves the physician to understand the basic principles involved in a biomechanical assessment, to eschew a too theoretical approach to mechanics, and to search for the practical applications. An understanding of the biomechanics of running facilitates this strategy.

The subtalar joint is a linchpin of the system of stress distribution. Its axis is triplanar, passing from posterior, lateral, and inferior to anterior, medial, and dorsal. It is also described as being a mitred hinge joint, reflecting its association with pronation/supination in the foot and internal/external rotation in the lower leg. Rear foot valgus is the hind foot position when the subtalar joint is everted. When combined with abduction and dorsiflexion in the foot pronation takes place. On the other hand, rear foot varus indicates inversion of subtalar joint that, when combined with abduction and plantar flexion, contributes to supination of the foot.

The neutral position of STJ is achieved when one-third of the movement from eversion to inversion has taken place, and is found at midstance in the halt cycle. The midtarsal joint comprises the talonavicular and calcaneocuboid joints, with motion occurring in all planes around longitudinal and oblique axes. A full range of motion at the midtarsal joint is dependent upon the 'unlocking' of the subtalar joint in pronation. Assessment of the position of the forefoot relative to the hindfoot in determines any degree or forefoot varus or vulgus.

The running-gait cycle includes phases of stance, float, swing, and further float. During the early stance phase the centre of gravity asses forward over the hindfoot, requiring a relative leg shortening. The STJ everts and the foot pronates. Transmission of force and motion to the midtarsal joints, and thence to the forefoot, allows the plantar surface of the forefoot to accommodate to te ground surface. Pronation is largely a passive event without muscular control. From midstance to toe-off supination takes place, during which both intrinsic and extrinsic foot muscles are active prior to the provision of heel-lift by the triceps surge. The limb then extends as the foot comes off the ground during acceleration.

Although the major it of long-distance runners use an initial heel-strike pattern, a small percentage have a midfoot strike. Sprinters usually have a forefoot strike pattern. The magnitude of the ground-reaction forces which occur during running may be measured by a force platform. Peak forces of three times bodyweight are seen.

Training schedules

Since inappropriate training schedules are a common source of overuse injury, it is clear that this is a subject with which the physician should be familiar. Naturally, a well-balanced training schedule is sought at all times, though the athlete recovering from injury is particularly at risk of relapse or further complications, unless muscle rehabilitation has been adequate and training is undertaken at the correct pace—that is, without abnormally large incremental increases in loading. His frustration during a period of disability and subsequently impatience to increase the intensity of training combine to cause further irritation if breakdown occurs. The physician may then be criticized for is 'mis-management' of te condition: indeed this may be a valid criticism if a suitable 'review' policy is not arranged on starting training. Particular care is required by the athlete at the beginning of a season and towards the close of the season. Overtraining may led to generalized fatigue and poor competitive performance. Serum creatine phosphokinase may be significantly raised both in over-training and in sports such as some martial arts, in which there is repetitive direct trauma.

The risk of injury may be lessened by increasing muscle strength. Studied of American university footballers, for instance, have demonstrated that te frequency ad severity of knee injuries are reduced by preseason to total-body conditioning. The importance of appropriate agnonist-antagonist balance or a particular sport, in addition to muscle power and endurance, cannot be overemphasized. Loss of sock-absorbing capacity may occur in fatigued muscles, thus leading to increased stress and microfractures in the area of bone adjacent to their attachments. Recurrent stress in musculotendinous units which are fatigued from repetitive eccentric contraction may result in tendinitis.

Common Traits

Athletes who have achieved the feeling of well-being or 'high' from the endorpin release associated with endurance exercise are not always able to adopt an analytical or sensible approach when setting themselves targets or goals. The type of exercise that in chosen in the pursuit of physical fitness or conditioning may be inappropriate. It is not always appreciated by the 'prospective athlete' that endurance exercise is required to attain the level of 'cardiorespiratory' fitness necessary for a healthy life-style. A schedule of thirty minutes of jogging, brisk walking, cycling, or swimming three or four times a week should be te goal for those seeking recreational rather that competitive activity. For those who expand their exercise programmes, the risk is the liner association between the intensity of endurance exercise and the indulgence of musculoskeletal injury.

Training Objectives

1. Flexible training

Adequate flexibility is essential for normal biomechanical function in sport. Performance may be compromised if flexibility is inadequate.

(a) Excessive muscle activity is require, leading to premature fatigue.

(b) Sports techniques are difficult, if not impossible, to achieve.

(c) Other training characteristics—for example, strength-training—may be impeded.

Of the factors affecting flexibility there are some which impose unyielding limitations—for instance, bone to bone, or bone to soft tissue impingement. But other factors, such as the following, may be influenced by flexibility exercises:

(a) the non-contractile structures that are an integral part of joints;

(b) the contractile structures that span joints.

The term laxity refers to the degree of passive distraction or shear of a joint in a specific direction: it results from ligamentous insufficiency, for instance medial laxity at the knee after MCL rapture. If mobility in a wide spectrum of joints is excessive, the term hypermobility is applied. Neither situation is desirable.

Muscles which are used repetitively and remain unstretched, or muscles which are trained for strength only, become shorter. However, viscoelastic forces allow muscles to achieve maximum force when initially stretched to approximately 120 % of their resting length. Thus to maximize the force required to kick a football the hip is initially extended, thereby stretching the rectus femoris, which is subsequently required as a power knee extensor. In throwing the javelin or discuss the trunk is rotated maximally, thereby stretching the pectoralls major, which contracts powerfully in the forward acceleration phase.

Flexibility training develops this capacity for viscoelastic energy storage by overload. Long slow stretching is required. Passive stretching is often reinforced with the aid of external forces, thereby creating passive 'assisted' stretching—for example, resting the heel of the outstretched leg on a plinth to stretch the hamstrings. Ballistic stretching, on the other hand, sold not be considered to be anything other than a form of 'toning up' for muscles. It stimulates the stretch reflex and, if equality, may provoke muscle pulls. De Vries found that flexibility may be improved significantly by both static and ballistic methods. Post-contraction relaxation is another technique that is utilized in both training and therapeutic contexts. Muscle may lengthen further after isometric contraction at the excrement of range—therapists use this principle in the technique of PNF.

In summary, flexibility exercises are used:

(a) in rehabilitation to re-establish normal joint function;

(ii) prophyiactically to prevent injury;

(iii) in training to achieve a maximally efficient biomechanical framework for specific sports technique.

2. Strength training

During strength training, or recovery from disuse atrophy, there is an increase in the number of muscle capillaries, an increase in myofibril size percell, and an increase in mitochondria. It is possible that interconversion between fibre type II-A and II-B is a response to training techniques. No such interconversion appears to occur between types I and II; selective recruitment of the different type II fibres appears to be the more logical response. Generation of new fibrils occurs, and must be given time between training sessions to compensate for fibril destruction. Thus it is important to allow at least twenty-four to forty-eight hours between sessions of intensive strength training. Application of heavy workload is necessary in strength training—and high-intensity low-repetition regimes are used. Increases in strength of up to 70 % are reported as typical training effects. However, endurance work requires repetitive stress with loads that correspond to 20-25 % of maximal capacity—that is, low-intensity high-repetition regimes.

Dynamic music activity is often a combination of isotonic contraction when muscle shortens, and isometric contraction when there is no change in length. Muscle may also contract eccentrically while lengthening. Visco-elastic energy is stored by muscle when pre-stretched or pre-loaded by eccentric contraction prior to concentric contraction. This principle is employed during a type of training known as plyometrics when various drills re used to develop power for running, jumping, and rowing. Such drills include hops, power bounds, depth jumps, and jumping with weights. Free weights, or throwing and catching a medicine ball, may be used for the upper body.

Progressive resistance training is the mainstay of the development of strength, power, and local muscle endurance. Gradually increasing overload must be applied to the musculoskeletal system as adaptation occurs. Relatively inexpensive equipment, in the form of barbells, dumb-bells, and ankle and wrist weights, relies on gravity for resistance. At no extra expense an athlete may utilize his own bodyweight for resistance, for instance in bench-stepping and press-ups, in a conventional 'circuit'. Multigyms usually rely on the gravity effects of stacked weights, though at somewhat greater cost. Sets of repetition are used, with the workload depending upon both the maximal capacity and te capability of the joint over which the muscle acts. Variation is required, as it has been observed that training by concentric contraction alone wiil not necessarily increase the ability to contract centrically.

Many both clubs and gymnasia now employ variable resistance, provided by equipment such as Nautilus or Atlanta. A series of cams and levers modifies the loading on a muscle at different angles of contraction. Although weight is selected in a similar way to the multi-gym, the engineering is such that ballistic movements are eliminated ad heavier weights are capable of being handled. In distinction from the situation fond using conventional weights, the athlete is not limited to using a weight that can be moved through the mechanically 'weakest' part of the muscle's range. The variable-resistance systems include a large number of pieces of equipment for exercising specific muscles or muscle-groups.

Isokinetic training employs a more specific 'accommodating resistance' by the use of hydraullics. a dynamometer offers an equal resistance as soon as the preset speed is reached, thus matching the muscle contraction. Increased muscular output produces increased resistance rather than the increased acceleration that would occur in gravity-loaded systems. Systems such as Cybex, Orthotron, and Lido include a compute linkage, so that torque in foot pounds and other measurement may be made. Peak torque is defined as the highest point on the generated torque curve in foot pounds. The joint angle at which peak torque occurs may be measured. A change in angular velocity affects this value: for instance, quadriceps peak torque occurs later in the range of motion with increasing speeds. Work, which is a reflection of the movement of force through a angular displacement, amy be measured, and is represented by the area under the torque curve. There is substantial evidence that isokinetic exercise increases the work that a muscle can do more rapidly than isometric or isotonic exercise

In comparing the mechanics of an isokinetic contraction with a dynamic one using weights as a resistance, the difference in the torque curve over the range of motion is striking. In an isokinetic exercise programme at the knee maximal resistance may be achieved throughout a complete range of motion. However, on examination of the torque values at 0° it may be seen that, if resistance work is required at or close to full knee extension, isometric training also should be employed.

Different sports require different muscles capabilities in respect of strength, power, and endurance. Eventually the establishment of a data base from testing protocols using isokinetic dynamometers should help to determine the function of specific muscle groups in each sport. Many sports, for instance soccer, demand a background of constant running interspersed with frequent demands for explosive power in the form of sort sprints. Weight-lifters also require power—that is, strong fast contraction. Therefore training should be appropriate, and include a full complement of exercise, not solely that designed for endurance. Pure endurance training reduces the strength and power of muscles. Any athlete who has experienced the difficulty in coping with the bursts of activity demanded in a game such as squash rackets after a period of long-distance running training will recognize this.

Fitness Assessment

1. Psychological assessment

Psychological factors have a significant effect on an athlete's capacity for training, and motivation for competition or increased intensity of effort. Factors which are generally believed to influence sports performance include anxiety, aggression, motivation, concentration, self-confidence, pain tolerance, and emotional state. Psychometric evaluation of abilities, aptitudes, and skills by objective measurement and techniques may be performed by the sports psychologist.

Yaffe used Nideffer's Test of Attention and Interpersonal Style to determine te capacity of talented young tennis players to cope with stress, and Eysenck's Personality Questionnaire to gauge sociability, impulsiveness, emotionality, and tough mindedness. Response to specific training and competitive situation is assessed by a structured interview.

2. Physiological assessment

The physiological components which may contribute to athletic performance may be outlined as follows.

(i) Physique. Whilst somatotyping individuals into ectomorphs, endomorphs, and the typically athletic mesomorph is interesting, it is of little practical benefit.

In sports such as American football it is quite clear that size is as important as explosive power. On the other hand, the variation in body size of 800 metre runners is quite extensive. The determination of body-fat per unit bodyweight is of more relevance, and may be calculated by te se of skin-calipers. Reference is made to conversion tables once average values are determined from the four skin-sites, i.e. those overlying triceps and biceps in the upper arm, at the inferior angle of the scapula, and finally over the iliac crest. Alternatively, lean bodyweight may be determined by electrical impedance.

(ii) Flexibility. Although an initial evaluation should be made during medical examination, the physiologist performs his own tests. The assessment of flexibility should not be confined to an isolated test for combined trunk flexion and hamstring elasticity, despite its relative importance. All the major joints are examined. Specific stretch tests for muscles which span two joints are performed. At very mobile joints range of motion in the position of function is recorded—for example, external rotation in 90° abduction of the shoulder in tennis players. Hypermobility should be recorded if present: it should be looked for routinely in dancers and gymnasts.

(iii) Muscle strength and power, Sheer 'strength' plays its part in a number of sports. It is usually required for limited periods—for example, in rugby scrummaging. The fast delivery of force—that is, of power which is measured in foot pounds or newton metres per second—is often much more relevant. Conventionally, when measured by an isokinetic dynamometer, the faster speeds—for example, 240° per 300° per second—are used, as it is thought that there more accurately reflect function. However, Rothstein et al. point out that no evidence exists to suggest that different speeds of movement test different muscular characteristics. Field tests such as sergeant jumps, short sprints, and throwing the sot in different ways offer a cruder indication of power in different muscle groups.

The Lido isokinetic dynamometer in use at the Sports ad Fitness Assessment Unit at the London Bridge Clinic has a number of practical applications in assessment and rehabilitation, summarized as follows:

(a) rehabilitation after injury;

(b) establishment of a data base of muscle function for fit individuals or team members;

(c) isokinetic training;

(d) determination of fatigue index—an anaerobic test of local muscle endurance;

(e) detection of muscle imbalance—as an assessment procedure or in established injury, for example, comparison of torque ratios of agonists and antagonists.

(iv) Anaerobic fitness. Explosive bursts of energy are required in a number of sports, and are provided by the creatine phosphate energy store and anaerobic glycolysis. An anaerobic test measures the quantities of work that a muscle group can produce maximally, in addition to its ability to recover. A typical example is the Wingate test using a cycle ergometer. Calculated values for the total work done and mean power output are measured for sort bursts of maximal exercise, and reflect the subject's work capacity. A recovery index may be determined by nothing the relevant recorded data on repeated tests after sort rest intervals. Alternatively, an isokinetic dynamometer may be used: the time taken for torque to drop to 50% of its initial value, or the torque level after 30 contractions at a high angular velocity, for example, 300° per second, are recorded. A fatigue index is determined by its means.

(v) Anaerobic threshold. At a given submaximal exercise intensity muscle relies largely on anaerobic metabolism to deliver energy. Much greater amounts are available, although for limited periods of time; the accumulation of chemicals such as lactic acid causes increasing discomfort. The anaerobic threshold depends on the body's capacity to metabolize lactic acid. Therefore determination of the AT yields information on the capacity to sustain high levels of aerobic work. When used to test endurance capacity it correlates better than max. Vo_{2}.

(vi) Aerobic fitness. The capacity of the cardiovascular system to deliver appropriate quantities of oxygen to working muscle is conventionally measured by determination of maximal O_2 intake. The Astrand method, depending on the use of conversion factors from a knowledge of heart rate and work performed, has been used for some time. A more accurate method requires expired air analysis, though increased costs may be restrictive. A sport-specific ergometer should be chosen if available—for example, bicycle, treadmill, rowing ergometer, or swimming flume. Gradually increasing effort to exhaustion is required of the athlete.

Max. Vo_2 should be measured in athletes whose sports involve over two minutes of continuous vigorous activity. Aerobic capacity depends on the ability of muscles to cope with the available oxygen. Muscular endurance as well as cardiovascular efficiency is improved by training. Max. Vo_2 in the relatively unfit may improve by up to 25% following suitable training. Typical figures in athletes who depend on high aerobic capacity are 65-80 ml per kg bodyweight.

Community Fitness

The need for a increased emphasis upon disease prevention within the framework of the National Health

Service in the UK has been appreciated for some time. Various arguments, not least those involving financial implications, have apparently prevented its more extensive development. Debate still continues over te relative importance of the aetiological factors implicated in the health scourge of affluent Western civilization—coronary carter atherosclerosis. There is general agreement over the adverse effects of smoking and hypertension, though the subsidiary roles of obesity, stress, and a sedentary existence seem less clear. Hypercholesterolemia appears to be involved, with the result that fat-reducing diets are widely available.

Studies have purported to show the usefulness of regular exercise in the prevention of progressive coronary artery disease after a first myocardial infarct. A logical extension of this argument is that exercise may prevent the initial onset of coronary artery disease in the asymptomatic subject, possibly by assisting in maintenance of serum cholesterol and weight within accepted norms. Although studies such as that by Morris et al. in London, Paffenbarger and Hale in San Francisco longsoremen have shown an association between active jobs and reduction in ischemic heart disease, a causal relationship is not established. Furthermore, comparison of the apparent beneficial effects of work activity and leisure pursuits is difficult. Nevertheless it is generally accepted that exercise reduces the likelihood of developing coronary heart disease. Morris et al. have shown that the important aspect of this cardio-protective effect is repeated bouts of vigorous exercise, rather than overall energy expenditure. Other benefits to health from exercise are as follows:

(a) facilitation of management of chronic disease such as diabetes;

(b) improvement of mood;

(c) prevention of osteoporosis;

(d) increase in physical working capacity.

Evaluation of risk factors is available at screening centres within the private medical sphere in the UK. The more dynamic aspects the private of health and fitness, with particular reference to the role of exercise, are determined by appropriate tests at the Sports and Fitness Assessment Unit at the London Bridge Clinic. The testing protocol conforms to as sophisticated a system of dynamic assessment as is currently available.

(1) Medical examination identifies abnormalities of the musculoskeletal system as well as other physiological systems. Flexibility is assessed. The resting blood pressure is measured.

(ii) Body fat percentage is calculated from skin caliper measurements.

(iii) Muscle power an endurance are assessed on a Lido isokinetic dynamometer.

(iv) Anthropometric measurements include height and weight.

(v) Urinalysis and hematological screening, including cholesterol and triglycerides, are undertaken.

(vi) Lung function is determined by spirometry.

(vii) Aerobic fitness is measured by expired air analysis, Maximal exercise testing using one of several protocols on a treadmill or bicycle ergometer is performed on subjects who take regular vigorous exercise. Max. Vo_2 and anaerobic thresholds are calculated, where possible, and assessment made by comparison with age-related tables. Submaximal tests are used for subjects who do to take regular exercise or who are recovering from cardiac disorders or bypass surgery: nevertheless max. Vo_2 may be computed from tabulated oxygen consumption. The test is concluded when the subject's heart rates rises to the target heart rate adjusted for age.

(viii) Cardiac function is assessed by a stress ECG using a 12-channel 12-lead Marquette machine while the subject exercises on a treadmill or cycle.

(ix) Finally a 'prescription' is issued with suggestions for a healthier life-style, including a suitable exercise regime. The subject's inclinations, musculoskeletal capabilities, and cardio-vascular tolerance are taken into account in the formulation of the prescription.

Exercise Prescription

Three components should be included.

(a) Warm-up. During this five-minute phase exercises to stretch large muscle-groups are performed, preparing them for sustained activity. The combination of long slow stretch and muscle-toning in the form of jogging on the spot or hopping increases muscle blood-flow.

(b) Cool down. During this phase body metabolism is allowed to return to normal gradually by the inclusion of a reduced level of muscle activity. Calisthenic exercises, which have the added desirable effect of improving anaerobic fitness, may be added to walking or a slow log.

(c) Endurance or aerobic. During this phase, lasting fifteen to thirty minutes, intensity should be tailored, depending upon the baseline of fitness, to increase aerobic capacity. Although different formulae are used, a rule of thumb guide is for a target heart rate of approximately 75% of maximal safe heart rate to be achieved and maintained. Maximal heart rate is usually considered to be 220 minus age. For example, for a forty-year-old 220 - 40 =180 beats per minute. Clearly the type of aerobic activity will depend upon a number of factors already outlined: fast walking, swimming, cycling, and jogging are commonly prescribed.

Injury Prevention in Children

An understanding of the pattern of musculoskeletal injury in children is required prior to a consideration of injury prevention. The different patterns of injury are dependent on the difference in the relative strength of the various component in the child compared with the adult. Thus indirect stress applied to the articular framework in children is more likely to result in epiphyseal fracture thin in ligament disruption. Salter and Harris classified fractures involving the epiphysis into grade I-V depending upon the extent of the involvement of the metaphysis or disaphysis. When faced with apparent joint injury in the child radiological investigation of the epiphysis should be undertaken, and orthopaedic surgical opinion should be south if disturbance is detected. Joint instability tends to be caused by avulsion of a bony fragment attached to a ligament, rather than to an intraligamentous tear. The equivalent of the anterior cruciate ligament tear in the adult is avulsion fracture of the inferior attachment of the ACL at the intercondylar area of the tibia. Surgical management by re-attachment of the bony fragment is advisable. In general a satisfactory outcome may be excepted following such fracture management.

Traction forces which result in muscle tear or tendon rupture in the adult tend to cause fracture separation of the apophysis in the child. Examples of acute avulsion fractures are found in the pelvic girdle. The affected apophyses are located at:

(i) lesser trochanter—insertion of iliopsoas.

(ii) anterior superior iliac spine—origin of sartorius.

(iii) iliac crest—origin of gluteus medius and

insertion of external oblique.

(iv) anterior inferior iliac spine—origin of hamstrings.

(v) ischial tuberosity—origin of hamstrings.

Fragmentation of an apophysis that results from chronic repetitive stress is referred to as a traction osteochnodrosis. Example of stress injuries to the apophyses in the upper limb and found at the coracoid process and in the lower limb at the tibial tubercle and the posterior calcaneal tubercle. The acute injuries should be treated in the same way as muscle tears—that is, with a full stretching and strengthening programme during rehabilitation. The stress injuries require reduction of load; relative rest for two to three months may be sufficient.

Overue injury patterns are similar to those in the adult. Stress fractures are common, though they may occur at the epiphyseal growth plate as well as he diaphysis. In the upper limb stress fractures of the proximal humeral epiphysis in Little Leaguers and of the distal radial epiphysis in gymnasts have been recorded. X-rays often show widening of the epiphysis: bone scans may confirm the diagnosis, though interpretation is sometimes difficult as there is increased uptake in the normal epiphysis. Stress fractures in the lower limbs conform to a similar pattern to those found in adults. Stress fractures in the partes interarticulares of the lower lumbar vertebrae are largely confined to children under twelve, when they are often relatively painless, and to adolescents, when they are usually painful. Repetitive micro-trauma may lead to compression fracture of the anterior margins of the vertebral bodies in he thoracic and thoracolumbar regions, giving rise to the clinical syndrome of Scheuremann's disease. A tight lumbodorsal fascia associated with an increased lordosis are thought to be contributory factors.

Disorders of the articular cartilage may also occur during growth spurts. Osteochondritis dissecans of the capitelum is seen in gymnasts., Osteochondritis dissecans of the knee occurs in juniors as well as in adolescents. Although the etiological factors remain unproven, recurrent microtrauma is suspected.

In the determination of the aetiological factors involved in overuse injury a full range of possible abnormalities of technique, malalignment, and abnormal biomechanics should be studied as for the adult. In some sports, such as swimming, the peak of potential may be realized while the child is still in the mid-teens. Miles of swimming training may be performed each day, resulting in injury to the shoulder, in particular, and to other areas, of which the most notorious is breast-stroker's knee. Other sports, including gymnastics and dance in its various forms, require training from an early age. Extreme flexibility is required in many joints. Injury patterns may be associated with lack of flexibility in crucial areas—for instance, inadequate hip mobility leading to low back injury in ballet dancers.

In some youngsters in their early teens recurrent injury may be associated with relative tightness of the musculotendinous structures. Growth spurts involve axial lengthening of the long bones. Unless flexibility exercises for the contractile tissues are undertaken at this time recurrent muscle pulls may be sustained. Usually the child is no more inclined than the average adult to perform regular stretching exercises, and therefore must be suitably encouraged.

6

CARE AND PREVENTION OF MUSCULO-SKELETAL INJURIES

It is usually observed that all injury leaves pain in the memory and for Olympic-calibre athletes, the memory often is not limited to the injury itself, but frequently includes the lifelong pain of lost opportunity. Injury can affect peak performance - through the loss of a millimetre or fraction of a second- and be the deciding factor in being chosen for an Olympic medal. As tragic as injury can be in denying an athlete the joy of Olympic competition, so too is Olympic history replete with stories of courageous athletes who have overcome injury to achieve the enduring glory of Olympic success.

Al Oerter, in Tokyo in 1964 won the third of his four gold medals by ignoring the pain of a dislocated cervical vertebra and torn rib cartilage and hurling the discus an Olympic record distance of 60.54m. In receiving his unprecedented third gold medal, Oerter said, these are the Olympics. You die for them.

Injury is an undeniable facet of athletic life. Individuals across the spectrum of competitive levels, from recreational athletes to Olympic competitors, are subject to the limitations and disappointments imposed by musculoskeletal injury. Elite athletes, however, are particularly susceptible to the physical, emotional and economic costs that injury exacts. Though these costs are in consequential for minor injuries, they can be overwhelming in cases of devastating injury that make it impossible, either temporarily or permanently, for an athlete to train and compete.

Lessening the chance of injury and facilitating the treatment and recovery of injured athletes requires and interdisciplinary approach that includes consideration of the anatomical, physiological, medical, kinesiological, psychological and mechanical aspects of athletes and their competitive environments. The injury-related problems of elite athletes are not addressed optimally by each discipline acting in isolation. The interdisciplinary team may include medical professional, physical therapists, athletic trainers, sport scientists, psychologists, coaches and athletes.

Each of these professionals brings a specific perspective to the challenges of dealing with injuries to athletes. In addition to these individual perspectives, musculoskeletal injury can be viewed from many different general perspectives, including historical, epidemiological, economic, psychological and biomechanical.

EPIDEMIOLOGICAL PERSPECTIVE

Epidemiology- the study of the incidence, distribution and control of disease and injury- documents the frequency and distribution of a particular injury in a given population. With the large number of participating nations, the huge array of sporting events and numbers of participating athletes, and the scatter in data-collection procedures, comprehensive injury data for Olympic athletes do not exist. While isolated reports of injuries to specific groups of Olympic competitors are available comprehensive documentation of injuries to Olympic athletes is unavailable and may remain so in light of the logistical constrained to gathering such data. In the general population, many injuries are never officially recorded. Thus published injury statistics are underestimates of the true injury toll. This is undoubtedly true for Olympic athletes as well; it is highly likely that many more injuries happen than are officially recorded and reported.

Historical Perspective

Archaeological evidence suggests that musculoskeletal injury is as old as itself. As well, injury is endemic to athletic lore, as illustrated in the legendary tale of Phidippides, who fell dead on the plain of Marathon after running 40 km and proclaiming the news of the Atheneum victory over the Persian forces of Dariuys the Great.

Injuries always have been and will continue to be a part of the athletic experience for participants at all level of sport. Despite the inevitability of injury, athletes have benefited greatly from medical progress in the 20th century. Advances such as clinical arthroscopy, pioneered by Bircher in the early 1900s, presaged an age in which rapidly developing technologies would render tractable many problems that were previously impossible to solve. Not long ago, laser surgery, advanced imaging techniques, micro- surgery and computer- or robot-assisted surgery were dismissed as futuristic dreams. Such medical advance, combined with remarkably improved rehabilitative programs, not provide new hope where previously there was only despair. Many athletes, who in earlier times would have been unable to compete due to injury, are now able to fulfil their dreams of Olympic participation.

Economic Perspective

While injury exacts physical and emotional coasts, the economic consequences of injury are often overlooked. Such costs include direct costs and morality costs. Since death due to athletic injuries is rare, the last of these costs is of minor consequence. The combination of direct and morbidity costs resulting from athletic injuries, however, is considerable. For an event such as the Olympic Games, these costs can account for a significant portion of the event's budget. At an individual level, the costs can be even more catastrophic, especially in cases where one's economic livelihood is predicated on his or her athletic success.

Psychological Perspective

The most noticeable consequence of injury is the direct, physical damage to the body's tissues. Less obvious, and arguably no less important, are the psychological consequences that accompany musculoskeletal injury. Injury-related psychological factors can be involved before, during and after the actual injury, and can influence the likelihood and severity of injury, and the course of treatment and rehabilitation.

The psychological profiles of highly competitive, Olympic-calibre athletes differ in many ways from those of the general population. Psychological attributes such as high motivation, pain tolerance, goal orientation and exemplar physical training habits can benefit one's performance. On the negative side, elite athletes may be predisposed to a higher sense of loss, greater threat to their self-image, and harbour unrealistic expectations and a desire for a quick recovery from injury. While some psychological factors are common to athletes across a wide range of athletic events, the risk of injury also is clearly event-dependent. An Olympic alone skier or boxer, is much likely to suffer an injury than a participant in events such as curling of archery. Psychological factors affecting athletic performance and injury should be neither underestimated nor ignored.

Biomechanical Concepts

Movement is inherent to life and the quintessential element of our being. Without movement there would be no life. Some forms of movement developed to ensure survival, and others evolved as a means of expression. Athletic movements, in particular, are among the most demanding of all those imposed on the human body's framework.

Assessment of movement from a descriptive perspective falls within the area of mechanics known as kinematics. Kinematic analysis of movement involves five -primary descriptive variables.

1. acceleration indicating how quickly the velocity has changed.

2. velocity measuring how fast something has moved.

3. displacement describing what movement has occurred;

4. position or location.

5. time temporal characteristics of movement.

Movement description provides a useful tool for coaches and athletes in assessing the movement demands of their respective sports. Description alone, however, has limitations, and a comprehensive analysis of a movement pattern or skill also requires knowledge of the forces that produce the movement. Analysis of the force-related characteristics of movement falls within the area of mechanics known as kinetics.

Biomechanical perspective

Off all scientific disciplines, physics and its subdiscipline, mechanics, are arguably most central to the study of injury, since most injuries have mechanically related causes. Forces and force-related factors are the prime agents that determine the likelihood and severity of injury. The nature of an injury and its treatment rests on the effective integration of biological and mechanical knowledge. Interdisciplinary biomechanics is ideally positioned to provide this integrated perspective. In the case of musculoskeletal injury to prevention, diagnosis and severity. The goal is to mitigate the negative effects of injury and allow athletes at all levels to maximize their performance potential.

Force and Pressures

Body movements are produced and controlled by forces acting both within the body and upon body from external sources. These forces, in addition to modulating movement patterns, also act on tissues in the body. Under most conditions, these forces are well tolerated by the body's tissues in the body. Under most conditions, these forces are well tolerated by the body's tissues. Indeed, force is central to optimal growth and development of tissues, especially those such as bone that provide structural support. But when forces exceed a tissue's ability to withstand the load, injury occurs. Force therefore is the most fundamental element in injuries.

Force is defined as the mechanical action or effect applied to a body that tends to produce acceleration.

The standard unit of force is the newton, which is defined as the amount of force necessary to accelerate a 1 kg mass at 1 m. Forces pertinent to injury analysis include those that act in or upon the human body, and include gravity, impact, musculotendinous forces, ligamentous forces that stabilise joints, and forces applied to bones. For all injury related forces, seven factors combine to determine the nature and severity of the injury. These factors

1. rate how quickly is the force

2. variability is the magnitude of the force or variable over the application interval?

3. duration over what time interval is the force applied?

4. direction where is the force directed?

5. location where on the body or structure is the force applied?

6. magnitude how much force is applied?

Injury often occurs when one object impacts with another, such as when an ice- hockey player collides with an opponent or with the boards. Impact also occurs when an object such as a ball contacts an athlete. A sharp object contacting the skin with a given force level will cause a different injury than a blunt object that impacts the skin with a similar force. In general, as the area of force application increases, the likelihood of injury decreases. This relation between force and application area is measured by pressure, which is defined as the applied force divided by the area over which the force is applied. The standard unit of pressure is the pascal, defined as 1 N force applied to an area m². In cases where forces are applied to structures over

t
s
to
pr
loac
mea:
princ
stres:
Tensil

Compressive strain produces a decrease in the longitudinal dimensions of a tissue, such as when a vertebra is subjected to a compressive load.

Biological tissues have complex relations between stress and strain. Skin deforms readily under relatively low forces, whereas bone develops considerable internal resistance and deforms little. The responses of connective tissues such as tendon, ligament and cartilage fall between these two extremes. The relation between stress and strain can be visualized by plotting stress as a function of strain. The ratio provides a single numerical value describing the relation between stress and strain. This ratio it termed the stiffness of the material. Bone is relatively stiff and deforms little as loads are applied; by comparison, tendon is less stiff than bone. Typically, the mechanical responses of biological tissues are not linear throughout their physiological ranges, as explained in the next section.

Modes of Loading

During athletic activities, body tissues are continuously subjected to forces that vary in magnitude, location, direction, duration, frequency, variability and rate. In most cases, the body tolerates these forces well, but when loads exceed the normal physiological range- a not uncommon occurrence in elite athletes- tissues can experience overload and sustain injury. Injuries resulting from a single or a few overload episodes are called acute injuries. These injuries often happen with a violent impact, such as when a downhill skier loses control and crashes into a restraining barrier.

Where repeated loading leads to tissue damage, the injury is called an overuse or chronic injury. Calcaneal tendonitis in a long-distance runner provides chronic, overuse injury. Distinguishing acute form chronic injuries usually poses little difficulty. However, a relation between the two types sometimes exists. Chronic loading may weaken a tissue and increase its susceptibility to injury. A runner with chronic inflammation of the calcaneal tendon, may be predisposed to acute rupture of that tendon.

Torsion

A twisted structure experienced torsional loading, when the lower twists during a rapid change of direction while the foot is planted on the ground. Anatomical structures in the lower leg visit the applied torsional load. The ability of a bone to resist these applied torques depends on the bone's structural integrity. Several important principles govern a bone's torsional resistance.

1. torsion produces tensile and compressive stresses in the form of helical stress trajectories, which are maximal at the bone's surface. Excessive torsional loading can result in spiral failure along these lines.

2. shear stresses develop across the bone's cross section.

3. the stiffer the material being loaded, the harder it is to deform.

4. the larger a bone's radius, the more resistance it develops and the more difficult it is to deform.

Bending

A long, slender structure can be viewed mechanically as a beam. Forces acting perpendicular to the long axis of the beam create bending. In bending, the concave surface of the bone experience compressive stress; the convex surface of the bone is subjected to tensile stress. The maximal stresses occur at the surface of bone, with lower stresses developed away from the surface towards the midline of the bone. The bone resists the bending moment created by external forces. Greater increases in bending loads can cause the bone to fail.

Axial Loading

The simplest form of force application is uniaxial loading. In this mode, forces act along a single line, most often along the primary axis of the structure, such as when a long bone is loaded in compression or a tendon is pulled in tension by the action of its skeletal muscle. The tissue's response varies with the direction of the load. As noted earlier, biological tissues can demonstrate linear behaviour through certain loading ranges. A generalized stress-strain curve is presented. As the stress increases, the tissue's behaviour changes from its initial linear response to a non-linear region beyond,

In the real world of the athlete, forces are not always uniaxial in nature. Forces are typically multi-dimensional. The concepts of stress and strain are still applicable, but they interact across more than one dimension and thus present a more complex response.

Mechanisms of upper-extremity injuries in athletes

Most Olympic events require athletes to perform upper-extremity movements, especially overhead movements involving lifting, throwing and striking. Among these are athletic field events such as the javelin, discus, shot put, hammer throw and pole vault, as well as weight-lifting, baseball, soft-ball, volleyball and water polo. Other events such as Nordic skiing, rowing, ice hockey and swimming involve repetitive upper-extremity movements that also may predispose athletes to injury. Instability of upper-extremity joints, in particular the shoulder, and the repetitive nature of the throwing and lifting events, often lead to overuse injuries. Several such conditions and their mechanisms of injury are detailed in the following sections.

Elbow Fracture / Dislocation

In contrast to the chronic, overuse injuries just described are acute injuries caused by the rapid application of large forces. At the elbow, such injuries usually manifest as fractures or dislocations. Given the elbow's relative stability, it is no surprise that the elbow is more than three times less likely than the shoulder to suffer dislocation. Elbow joint luxation usually is accompanied by extensive soft-tissue damage that includes complete rupture or avulsion of both the ulnar and radial collateral ligaments. The elbow's bony configuration provides considerable resistance to anterior dislocation. As a result, most elbow dislocations occur posteriorly. The most common mechanics involves axial compressive forces applied to an extended or hyperextended elbow, such as would happen when someone falls onto an extended or hyperextended elbow, such as would happen when someone falls onto an extended arm. The forces in this position lever the ulna out of the trochea and rupture the capsule and ligaments, and thus allow joint dislocation.

Elbow fractures can happen to any of the three bones comprising the joint and are determined by the nature, magnitude, location and direction of the applied forces. Fracture of the distal humerus can occur in any area of the bone, including the supracondylar, intercodylar, condyle, epicodylar and articular regions. Ulhar fractures commonly involve the olecranon process, and may be caused by either direct and violent insult to the elbow joint through the forearm. Radial head fractures typically result from axial of the radius during a fall.

Musculoskeletal injuries, while an unfortunate fact of life for everyone, have special urgency for athletes, especially those committed to competing at the highest levels. Regrettably, many athletic careers have been appeared or even ended by injury. Olympic-level athletes often depend on precise upper-extremity movements for success in their sport or event. Compromised upper-extremity function caused by injury, however slight, can have profound repercussions in the athlete's performance. A clear understanding of the mechanisms of musculo-skeletal injury can aid in the effective diagnosis and treatment of the athlete, and a knowledge of injury mechanisms also may lead to better injury prevention strategies- the best injury is the one that never happens.

Valgus-Extension Mechanism

Medial epicondylitis and other injuries affecting the elbow often result from movement patterns involving throwing. Numerous studies have explored the kinematics and kinetics of the elbow during the throwing motion, which typically is divided into five phases; windup, cocking, acceleration, deceleration and flow-through. Several of these studies quantified elbow kinetics and found large and potentially injuries forces and moments. Near the end of the cocking phase, the elbow experience valgus loading as the elbow approaches terminal extension. This valgus loading is resisted by a varus torque produced by musculotendinous and particular tissues. Varus torques at this time have been estimated at between 64 and 120 Nm, with an associated joint force of about 500 N between the humerus and radius.

The coupled effect of valgus torque and elbow extension produces a valgus-extension mechanisms that can overload the joint and lead to medial elbow injuries such as epicondylitis, ulnar collateral ligament rupture, avulsion fracture and nerve damage.. The valgus stress also causes compression of the lateral radio-capituopitular joint and impingement of the medial aspect of the olecranon on the olecranon fossa. Repeated impingement leads to inflammation and eventual osteophyte formation on the posteromedial aspect of he olecranon process.

In throwing, as in other dynamic movements, the highest loads occur during phases when eccentric muscle actions are required to control high-velocity motion. Repeated development of such large loads can lead to progressive tissue degeneration that culminates in failure. This process is common but not inevitable. Some athletes are able to accommodate large, repeated loads with little, if any, symptomatic response. The answer remains elusive as to why some athletes are susceptible to overload injuries while others apparently are unaffected.

Epicondylitis

Most elbow injuries result from overuse and are characterized by progressive tissue degeneration that begins with asymptomatic microtrauma and evidence of intracytoplasmic calcification, collagen fibre splitting and kinking, and abnormal fibre cross-links. Continued loading exacerbates the tissue damage and leads to symptomatic inflammation, inflexibility, and tissue weakness.

The specific dynamics of an athletic task determine whether epicodylitis affects the medial or lateral aspect of the elbow. In tennis, the lateral epoicodyle experiences injury five times as often at the medial side. Lateral epicondylitis is most commonly attributed to inflammation of the proximal attachment of the extensor carpi radialis brevis during execution of the backhand stroke.

When a player strikes the ball, forces are generated in the wrist extensor muscles. These loads are transferred through the stiffened forearm musculature to the proximal attachment on the lateral humerus. Medial epicodylists happens much less frequently in tennis players and is due largely to extreme forces developed during the forehead and service strokes when the eccentric action of wrist flexors is required to control wrist extension. In cases of both medial and lateral epicondylitis, the suspected injury mechanisms include poor stroke mechanics, off-centre ball contact with the racket, grip tightness, wrist position at contact, and racket vibration.

Lateral epicondylitis is not exclusive to tennis. Athletes in other sports that involve backhand striking movements also are susceptible a chronic pathologies of the lateral elbow. Though less common, medial epicondylitis afflicts athletes across a wide range of sports, including archery, baseball, weight-lifting, javelin, handball, swimming and racquetball.

These sports involve repetitive upper-extremity movements that predispose the athlete to overuse. The forearm muscles pose fatigue and the resulting muscle weakness leads to eccentric failure of the flexor-pronator mass. The confluence of this group's muscle attachments on the medial epicondyle is subjected to repetitive microtrauma and subsequent inflammations. Athletes affected by medial epicondylitis often are aggressive players participating at elite levels who subject their elbows to extraordinary stresses.

Elbow Injuries

The elbow provides the critical middle link in the kinetic chain of the upper extremity. It is a synovial hinge joint formed by the dual articulations of the capitulum of the humerus with the head of the radius and the trochlea of the humerus with the trochlear notch of the ulna. Normal elbow motion is limited to uniplaner flexion-extension, with forearm pronation-supination produced by concurrent rotation of the proximal and distal radio-ulnar joints. The elbow is reinforced by collateral ligament complexes on the medial and lateral aspects of the joint. Elbow flexion is controlled by concentric action of the biceps branchii, branchialis and brachioradialis, with joint extension controlled by the triceps brachii.

Before considering mechanisms of elbow injury, we note several catch-all terms used to describe elbow injuries. The most common of these is tennis elbow, a term with various meanings ranging from a general descriptor of elbow pain to a specific reference to lateral epicondylitis. As with this and other nebulous terms, we discourage their use and prefer instead to use specific clinic descriptors.

Rotatory Cuff Pathologies

Rupture of musculotendinous structures in the

rotator cuff is the final step in a chain of events that has been described as an instability continuum. The progressive pathologies of instability, subluxation and impingement lead ultimately to rotator cuff tearing in some athletes. While not common in younger athletes, rotatory cuff tears can significantly affect an athlete's ability to train and perform. The loading characteristics of the rotator cuff depend on the functional demands of an athlete's sport or event.

Each sport has its own specific demands. Electromyographic data show that rapid and precise movement patterns elicit selective muscle action and periods of high muscle intensity. In spite of the unique phasic patterns particular to each throwing or striking sport motion, there is general pattern common to most. Perry described this common pattern as starting with a gentle approach to an appropriate starting position, followed by a cocking phase in which shoulder structures are tensed to provide a forceful acceleration.

Once the necessary acceleration has been accomplished, the system's muscles typically act eccentrically to decelerate the arm to avoid injurious forces. Repetitive attempts to decelerate the horizontal adduction, internal rotation, and glenohumeral distraction forces during the deceleration phase of throwing can lead to an eccentric tensile overload failure of the rotator cuff muscles, especially the supraspinatus. Repeated movements also can lead to muscle fatigue and compromised tissue integrity that contribute, in turn, to altered movement mechanics. Modifications in movement control and technique can further stress the tissues and hasten additional damage and eventual failure.

As noted, the supraspinatus is the most frequently injured muscle of the rotator cuff group and is most often associated with repeated, and often violent, overhead movement patterns. The other rotatory cuff muscles, while less susceptible to injury, are not immune to injury.

The muscles involved depend in part on the movement pattern and the task demands placed on the shoulder. Burkhart described four patterns of rotator cull kinematics associated with specific cult lesions. Type 1 lesions exhibited tears of the supraspinatus and portions of the infraspinatus, but not to an extent that disrupted essential mechanical force couples. Patients in this group had normal motion and near-normal strength.

Patients with Type-II lesions had massive teras of the superior and posterior portions of the rotator cuff. These resulted in an uncoupling of the essential force couples and led to an unstable fulcrum for glenohumeral motion. Type II patients were extremely limited and could do little more than through their shoulders.

Type III pathologies had partial tears of the subscapularis accompanying supraspinatus and major posterior cuff lesions. These injuries prevented the muscles from centering the humeral head in the glenoid fossa did led to superior humeral subluxation. Type IV lesions involved tears of the subscapularis and supraspinatus with no involvement of the posterior cuff muscles.

The complex shoulder movements required in many sports place considerable stress on the muscles of the rotatory cuff group. The throwing motion, in particular, places extraordinary loads on the shoulder. Throwing involves considerable abduction and external rotation of the arm, a position that places the rotator cuff at risk of injury, since high supraspinatus forces have been reported with the arm in the position. Those loads place the rotator cuff muscles at particular risk of injury. The role of the rotator cuff in synergistically resisting distraction of the humeral head is compromised by injury or fatigue to any of these muscles. The resulting alterations in throwing mechanics increases the likelihood of further tissue damage.

Impingement Syndrome

Much of the interest in glenohumeral impediment was stimulated by the pioneering work of Neer, who proposed an anatomical rationale and surgical treatment for chronic sub-acromical impingement syndrome. Glenohumeral impingement generally refers to arm abduction that results in the forcible pressing of supra-humeral structures, subacromial against the anterior surface of the acromion and the coracoacromial ligament that forms the coracoacromial arch. Repeated abduction impose large stresses on the capulogigamentous and musculotendinous structures of the glenohumeral joint. These stresses typically lead to tissue microtrauma, which with continued mechanical insulate can lead to tissue failure. Tissue failure then exacerbates joint instability and greater humeral movement. This, in turn, further aggravates the impingement condition. The athlete therefor is trapped in a negative feedback loop of compromised tissue integrity and joint function.

Impingement pathologies have been divided broadly into two age-related categories. Older individuals are most disposal to degenerative processes that promote bene spur formation, capsular thinning, decreased tissue perfusion, and muscle atrophy. More relevant to athletes is the second category, which includes individuals under 35 years who engage in sports involving extensive and repetitive overhead movements. Jobe and Pink proposed a classification system based on age related differences.

1. Group I injuries includes those of isolated impingement with no instability. This group typically includes older recreational athletes and only rarely includes younger athletes.

2. Group II patients exhibit instability with impingement secondary to overuse-related tissue microbrauma. This group comprise mostly young overhead athletes.

3. Group III injuries are closely associated with Group Ii pathologies common in younger athletes and are characterized by generalized ligamentous laxity and resultant shoulder instability.

4. Group IV includes injuries resulting from a traumatic event such as direct impact of a fall. Injuries in this group shoe shoulder instability without impingement.

The mechanisms of glenohumeral impingement remain controversial. The precise role of extrinsic intrinsic. Among the contributing factors are: the structural characteristics of the subacromial space 'the presence of bone spurs that focus forces on the subacromial structures and produce a functionally smaller supraspinatus outlet; degenerative processes affecting the supraspinatus; eccentric overload of the supraspinatus; muscular fatigue, compromised blood flow in regions of impingement pressure and relative tissue avascularity; and thickening of the coracoacromical ligament.

The risk factors for impingement closely parallel the movement characteristics of sports with extensive upper-extremity involvement. These include heavy work, direct load bearing, repetitive arm movements, working with hands above shoulder height, fatigue resulting from lack of rest, and high-velocity movements.

Impingement syndrome is not restricted to the general athletic population but afflicts special population athletes as well. Wheelchair athletes, suffer a high incidence of rotator cuff impingement pathologies. Burnham et al. reported that paraplegic athletes demonstrated an imbalance of abduction/adduction strength with relative weakness of shoulder adduction. In addition, paraplegics, shoulders affected by, impingement syndrome exhibited significant weakness of adduction, external and internal rotation when compared to the uninvolved shoulders. The suggested that strengthening of shoulder adduction and internal and external rotation may be an important prevention strategy for these athletes.

Glenohumeral Instability

A joint's ability to resist laxation is directly related to its inherent structural stability. The glenohumeral joint is strengthened by ligaments and surrounding musculature including the superficial deltoid and the deeper muscles of the rotator cuff. The glenoid labrum also contributes to joint stability, to a limited degree, by increasing the surface area and deepening the fossa, and thus improving the joint's bony fit. In spite of these supporting structural elements, the glenohumeral joint remains the least stable joint is the body, a distinction substantiated by its frequent dislocation. Simply stated, what the glenohumeral joint gains in mobility, it sacrifices in stability.

At the extremes of glenohumeral joint movement, such as at the end of the cocking phase in throwing, tension in the capsulo-gigamentous structures provides resisted to dislocation. During normal ranges of motion, however, laxity in these structures precludes their involvement in stabilizing the joint to a large extent. Other mechanisms are therefore needed to ensure joint stability. These mechanisms include limited joint volume, negative intra-articular pressure, concavity compression, and scapulohumeral balance.

In a normal shoulder with an uninjured joint capsule, a small negative intracapsular pressure contributes to joint stability. While not particularly large, this negative pressure nonetheless helps stabilize the glenohumeral articulation. Concavity compression- the stability created when a convex object is pressed into a concave surface- also contributes to joint stability. The surface of the humeral head and the glenoid fossa are pressed together by multiple muscle forces.

This pressure provides greater resistance to translational movement between the surfaces. Translational resistance in the glenohumeral joint is greater in the superior inferior direction than in the anterior-posterior direction and increases with greater compressive loading. Despite the resistance provided by concavity compression, translation of the humeral head on the glenoid fossa will happen with the combined movements of glenohumeral horizontal abduction and external rotation associated with the cocking phase of throwing.

These translational movements are relevant to skill mechanics since they indicate that the glenohumeral joint does not function purely as a ball-and-socket mechanisms but allows for anterior humeral head movement during glenohumeral flexion and cross-body movements and posterior translation with extension and external rotation.

Scapulohumeral balance describes the coordinated action of muscles controlling movement of the glenohumeral joint. The muscles most immediately responsible for maintaining scapulohumeral balance are those of the rotatory cuff group. The rotatory cuff muscles are assisted by action of the deltoid, latissumus dorsi, trapezius, serratues anterior, rhomboids and levator scapulae. To maintain joint stability, the net joint reaction force created by the combined action of these muscles must remain within the glenoid fossa. When muscle forces are uncoordinated, the joint reaction force may bot be balanced within the glenoid fossa and thus contributes to joint instability. Fatigue in any of the muscles compromises the ability of the musculoskeletal system to effect proper movement mechanics.

Glenohumeral instability predictably contributes to increased potential for other pathological shoulder conditions. Kvitne and Jobe described the progressive pathology of the overhand throwing athlete along a continuum from overuse inflammatory conditions to mild joint laxity with anterior subluxation, to internal impringement syndrome, and finally to rotatory cuff tearing.

Throwing athletes require sufficient joint flexibility

to achieve the joint ranges of motion required to generate high velocities. An athlete with inadequate flexibility may be advised to focus on increasing range of motion through appropriate stretching and strengthening exercises. On the other hand, repeated throwing can lead to increased joint laxity and range of motion. Brown et al., found that professional baseball pitchers exhibited 9^0 more external rotation in adduction in their dominant arm compared with the non-dominant side.

Such increases in range of motion, conceivably, could facilitate throwing performance, but more is not necessity better. Too much flexibility is detrimental since excessive stretching may enhance capsular laxity and lead to eventual shoulder instability.

Soft tissue adaptations may not be solely responsible for joint laxity. Recent evidence suggests that bony adaptations also may play a role in anterior glenohumeral instability. Pieper examined the degree of humeral retrogression in a group of male professional handball players, and found that the retrotosial angle of the humerus in a player's throwing arm was an average of 9.4° larger in the dominant side than in the non-dominant. Even more interesting form an injury perspective was the fact that in players without chronic shoulder pain, the side-to-side difference was 14.4° greater in the throwing arm. Players with chronic shoulder pain actually, showed a decrease of 5.2° of humeral retrogression in their throwing arm compared to the non-throwing arm. Piepere explained during growth to the repetitive external rotation demands of throwing practice. He concluded that Athletes who do not adapt this way seem to have more stain on their anterior capsules at less external rotation and development chronic shoulder pain because of anterior instability.

As noted previously, the glenohumeral joint is susceptible to luxation or subluxation. In rare cases, individuals with congenitally lax shoulders may experience a traumatic glenohumeral luxations. Most cases of shoulder dislocation, however, result from traumatic forces applied directly or indirectly of the glenohumeral complex. Ninety percent of more of glenohumeal luxations happen anteriorly, usually as a result of indirect axial forces applied to an extended, abducted and externally rotated arm. These forces effectively drive the humeral-head out of its normal position in the glenoid fossa. Much less frequently, anterior glenohumeral luxations is caused by direct forces applied to the posterior aspects of the shoulder.

Mechanisms responsible for the much less common posterior luxation basically are the reverse of those causing anterior dislocation. Indirect forces transmitted through a flexed, adducted and internally rotated arm, as would be seen in landing during a forward fall, effectively during the humerus posteriorly. Posterior luxation also can result from direct trauma applied to the anterior aspect of the humerus.

Shoulder Injuries

The shoulder joint is the upper extremity's most proximal articulation and influences most movements distal to it. Efficient upper extremity throwing and lifting skills depend on adequate glenohumeral joint range of motion and neuromuscular coordination. Shoulder injury usually precludes normal movement not only of the glenohumeral joint, but also of the elbow and wrist joints, especially in multi-joint movements.

Anatomically, the glenohumeral joint is formed by the articulation of the head of the humerus with the shallow glenoid fossa of the scapula. This loose fit of the humeral head within the glenoid fossa permits considerable triplanes movement, but also contributes to the least stable joint in the body.

Injury Mechanisms

Before examining the mechanics of specific musculoskeletal injuries, two terms required definition. The first is injury, defined as the damage sustained by tissues of the body. The second is mechanism, which is the fundamental physical process responsible for a given action, reaction or result.

Injury mechanisms are categorized according to mechanical concepts, tissue responses, or a combination of the two. The variety of injury types suggests a wide array of injury mechanisms. No single list or categorization system of mechanisms can adequately cover all types of injuries. Two exemplar classification systems, however, provide representative lists of injury mechanisms. Leadbetter listed contact or impact, dynamic overload, overuse, structural vulnerability, inflexibility, muscle imbalance and rapid growth as mechanisms of injury.

7

CARE AND PREVENTION OF SHOULDER INJURIES

Anatomy & Structure of Shoulder

Soft Tissue

The shoulder joint is enclosed in very loose capsule, or retaining bag of tissue, which covers the whole of the round head of he arm-bone, and attaches it to the outer rim of the receiving surface on the shoulder-blade. The capsule is thickened into protective ligaments over the front of the shoulder, but the joint's main protection is given by the tendons which cross the joint over its back, top and front. Your biceps tendon, which crosses the front of your shoulder, actually passes through the joint structure, adding another stabilizing force to the joint. The least protected part of the joint is its underside, in your armpit. When your arm is by your side, the joint capsule folds downwards in a loose pouch. When you lift your arm sideways, this slack is taken up, and the capsule is put on the stretch, but there are no thickened bands of ligaments or tendons limiting this movement or protecting the joint from excessive strain in this direction.

The soft, rounded contour of your shoulder is formed by the deltoid muscle, which spreads right over the front, back and top of he joint. This large muscle makes it difficult to feel the smaller structures lying closer to the joint.

Separating the tendons round the shoulder from each

other and from the joint structure are numerous bursae, or fluid-filled sacs. These provide friction-free movement between the tendons and the underlying tissues.

Pain in the Shoulder

A gradual pain in one or both shoulders can have a variety of causes. To help your doctor diagnose it accurately, you have to record exactly when the pain came on; what you were doing when you first felt it; whether it hurts at night or when you are resting; whether it gets worse or eases according to identifiable causes; whether it only comes on during or after sport, or whether you feel the pain at other times. Shoulder pain can be caused by an inflammatory arthritis or joint disease. It can also be referred from other parts of your body, for instance from a neck problems giving referred symptoms into the shoulder, or from a condition affecting your diaphragm, your main breathing muscles. Although you might feel the pain was specifically in your shoulder joint, there might be nothing wrong with the joint at all. One of the more serious problems which can cause shoulder pain is a heart condition, and sometimes your first warning of a heart problem is a pain which comes on, without a recognizable cause, in your left shoulder.

Bones

The shoulder is a ball-and-socket joint, formed between the side of your shoulder-balde and the top of your arm-bone. The shoulder-blade forms a flattened, circular disc opposite the top of the arm-bone, and this disc is made into a cup-shape by a ridge of soft-tissue all round its edge. The top of the arm-bone is rounded, conforming to the receiving surface on the shoulder-blade. But the two bones are not tightly bound together, and the front surface over the top of the arm-bone is much larger than the receiving surface at the side of the shoulder-blade. This means that the shoulder joint is quite different from the hip joint, although the two are parallel in structure, both being ball-and-socket joints, and both linking the limbs to your trunk.

Over the top of the shoulder you have an arch of bone which is separate from the shoulder joint structurally, but functionally linked to it. The acromion process is a wedge of bone at the end of the spine of the shoulder-blade, a ridge which you can feel clearly across the back of your shoulder. The acromion forms the hard tip you can feel over the top of your shoulder, and it joints onto the end of your collar-bone, just above the front of the shoulder. The spine of the shoulder-blade and the collar-bone form a V-shape, with the point of the V over your shoulder.

As the shoulder is padded with tick muscles, it is hard to feel the bones forming the joint. There are also a lot of nerves crossing the joint, which make it uncomfortable to press too hard over the bones. If you put your hand round the top of your arm-bone, so that your thumb is in your armpit, and lift your arm out sideways, you can feel the rounded end of the arm-one with your thumb, if you move your elbow backwards and forwards.

Functions

Your shoulder is the most mobile joint in your body. You can lift your arm forwards, backwards, sideways, and above your head. Your shoulder also twists, allowing you to place your hands behind your head or back. By combining all the available movements at the joint, you can achieve a full circular swinging movement, called circumduction, at the shoulder.

When you lift your arm straight out sideways, you can see your bulky deltoid muscle contract to produce the movement, and you can feel the muscle working if you put your hand over it. If you then take your arm forwards, keeping your elbow up in the air, you can feel the front part of your deltoid working over he front of your shoulder. If you swing your arm backwards with your elbow help up, you can feel the back portion of your deltoid contracting. When you hold your arm at your side, with your elbow bent to a right angle, and press your hand inwards towards your stomach against an immovable resistance, you can feel the rotator muscles on the front of your shoulder working isometrically. If you press your hand away from your body against a resistance, with your elbow bent, you can feel the contraction of the rotator muscles on the back of the shoulder, if you put your other hand over your shoulder.

In most movements of your shoulder, there is a complex interaction between the working muscles contracting and relaxing to produce the very wide range of movement possible. The shoulder joint does not work in isolation when you move your arm. The whole shoulder girdle has to move in harmony, so any arm movements involve not only the shoulder, but a movement of the shoulder-blade relative to the back of your ribs, and a less distinct, but important, movement in the joints between your collar-bone and of the breast-bone and acromion process at either end of it. If you stand with your back to a mirror, and look over you shoulder, you can see your shoulder-blades moving forward round your chest as you straighten your arms in front of you. Your shoulder-blades slide backwards towards your spine as you bring your arms back behind you, extending your shoulders.

The combination of power and mobility of power and mobility in your shoulder allows you to throw forcefully, so you can project a shot or discus, and bowl hard and fast in cricket. The service and smash strokes in tennis take your shoulder through a full arc, twisting the joint as you turn the racket behind your neck, then exerting a powerful thrust through the joint as you strike the ball. In combat sports, your shoulder mobility allows you to reach in various directions to grasp or hit your opponent. In judo and wrestling, shoulder lower lets you pull or push your opponent down.

Your shoulder can withstand strong forces which tend to pull it apart, or distract it. In gymnastics, hanging from the rings or high bar pulls the shoulder apart through the drag of your body-weight plus the effect of gravity. Because of the great mobility in your shoulders, you can do the so-called 'dislocation' movement, swinging your body in complete arcs, while you hold the bar or rings, keeping your hands a fixed distance apart. Your shoulders can also withstand great compression forces. When you do a hand-stand, your shoulders support your body-weight plus the effect of gravity. A single hand-stand places the total load through one shoulder. Power-lifters similarly support large compression forces through their shoulders when they lift weights overhead in snatch or press exercises.

Shoulder Injuries

Strains

The muscles and tendons over the shoulder can be injured by wrenching and twisting strains, by over-stretching and overuse, and by a forceful block to a movement while the muscles are contracting. The damage may be sudden and traumatic, or gradual and progressive.

Traumatic injuries to the shoulder may occur in contact and combat sports, riding, gymnastics and diving. You may fall awkwardly onto your hand or elbow, stretching your shoulder. An opponent may knock your arm, for instance in a rugby tackle, or block your throw in basketball. You may over-balance while doing a hand-stand in gymnastics. Overuse injuries are normally associated with sports in which you use your shoulder repetitively or continuously. Competitive swimmers produce about eighty percent of their stroke power through their arms, and their arduous training may overwork the shoulder muscles and tendons. An extra long, or unaccustomed, training session of tennis serving, shot putting, archery, or cricket bowling, may similarly over-strain the muscles and tendons, which become inefficient through fatigue.

What has happened?

In this type of injury, you strain or partly tear some muscles or tendon fibres in the affected area. You may also damage some of the ligaments protecting your shoulder. If you continue with your sport, and feel pain over the injury, you will do further damage to the injured tissues. If you use your shoulder awkwardly, trying to avoid hurting it, you will suffer from an almost immediate weakening in the muscles which are no longer being worked normally. The shoulder then loses the stability it owes to those muscles, and with this, its normal function and range of movement. This in itself sets up a cycle of progressive weakness and associated pain.

What you feel?

In a traumatic injury, you feel a sudden pain over your shoulder, which may be severe. You probably have to stop your sport, although, if it is a very minor injury, you may find that the pain subsides quickly and allows you to finish your game or session. In a gradual, overuse injury, the pain is usually only very sight to begin with.

You fee it on specific movements at the shoulder, and it gradually gets worse, if you continue to do your sport.

In either case, once the damage has occurred, you feel that pain whenever you move your shoulder, making the injured muscle or tendon contract or stretch out. You may be able to feel a tender spot where the tissues are injured, if you press over your shoulder with your other hand, although the bulk of your deltoid muscle makes it difficult to feel some of the individual tendons lying under its thickest parts. If the injury is over the front of your shoulder, contracting the muscles and tendons to take your arm forward, or turn it inwards, causes pain, and you feel a pull when you take your arm backwards and stretch the same muscles and tendons. An injury to the muscles and tendons at the back of the shoulder causes pain when you contract the muscles to take the arm backwards, or turn it outwards, or when you stretch them as you take your arm forwards. An injury to the deltoid muscles over the top of the shoulder is painful if you take your arm out sideways against a resistance.

Self-help measures for shoulder strains

(i) First-aid for the traumatic shoulder injury consists of ice application, and, if the pain is severe, support in a sling. You should then go as quickly as possible to the local casualty department or your doctor, for an assessment of the extent of the damage. It may be necessary for X-rays to be taken, if there is a risk that you might have cracked or broken one of the bones at the shoulder.

(ii) While your shoulder in painful, you should not try to continue with your sport, and you should try to avoid ay painful movements, while exercising the hoping specifically as much as possible. Once you have regained full flexibility in the injured muscles, and your shoulder feels strong because of the strengthening exercises, you can progress to the more demanding functional strengthening exercises, starting with a few at a time, and gradually increasing the amount you do. You must remember to maintain flexibility by stretching your shoulder muscles before and after any strengthening session.

(iii) When you start the stretching the exercises, you should also begin to do isometric and strengthening exercises, but avoiding ay exercises which cause pain. Choose up to six exercises, and do them once or twice a day, as time permits. If you can, it is best to do exercise in front of a mirror, to stop yourself 'cheating', by bending your trunk instead of using your shoulder.

(iv) When you are confident that you can do the functional exercises without pain, you can gradually resume your sport. Recovery from a shoulder strain may take only a week to ten days, if the injury was minor, and you started the rehabilitation process quickly. However, if you do not make sure that you have stretched and strengthened the joint thoroughly following the injury, you risk having niggling recurrences for a long time after the original injury, or, worse, you may find that your shoulder gradually stiffens up, while becoming weak, so that after a few months you have a real functional disability. Recovery after a severe injury may take six weeks or longer. Your guide to progress is any pain you feel, or your increasing ability to use your shoulder normally. If you do suffer from increasing ability to use your shoulder normally. If you must refer back to your doctor for further checks, to assess what is causing the setbacks, and whether there might be any complications underlying your shoulder pain.

(v) As soon as the acute pain subsides, your specialist

will probably advise you to start remedial exercises. If a specific muscle or tendon has been diagnosed as strained, you will start with gentle passive stretching exercises for the muscle group. If the injury is at the front of the shoulder, you do the exercises which take the arm backwards, creating a 'pulling' sensation over the joint. For an injury at the back of the shoulder, you do the exercises which pull the arm forward. What you should feel when you do the exercise is a slight pulling feeling over the injured area, and you hold this stretch position absolutely still for a count of ten. You should repeat the stretching exercises about three times every hour, if you possibly can, or do at least six stretching exercises twice a day, if you do not have time to do more.

(vi) For the overuse injury, you should refer to your doctor as soon as possible after you become aware of the pain, so that he can make an accurate diagnosis of the problem. If the pain has become severe, you can safely apply ice to soothe it.

Bursitis

The shoulder has many large bursae for friction-free movement between the tendons and their underlying tissues. Any of these bursae may become inflamed, either because you have been using your shoulder awkwardly during some activity, or as the result of an injury to a tendon or one of the other joint structures, which has caused irritation over the bursa.

An inflamed bursa causes pain whenever your shoulder moves in such a way as to catch the bursa or iritae it. Bursitis over the top of the shoulder causes pain when you stretch your arm out sideways, and when you twist it, especially inward, turning your palm down. Bursitis at the back of the shoulder causes pain when you twist your arm in either direction. Your may also be aware of a 'snapping' feeling at a particular point in your shoulder movement.

It is difficult for you to differentiate between the pain of bursitis and that caused by a muscle or tendon strain. The main difference is that the muscular strain gives pain when the muscle is worked or stretched, whereas the bursitis is painful in relation to shoulder movement, even when this is done in a completely relaxed way, for instance, if you let your arms swing drifting over the water surface in a swimming pool. The strained tendon or muscle may be painful in different ways, according to the position of your arm when the tissues are worked or stretched, and the amount of load the muscle or tendon works against when it is contracting. The bursitis may be getting more sharply painful, if the condition is getting worse, but you always feel its pain in the same place, whenever the bursa is caught in a position that irritates it.

You must avoid any painful movements, for a period of two to three weeks, to allow the inflamed bursa to ease. Your doctor may give you anti-inflammatory injections or tables to help the healing process. It is essential that you do not re-start your sport too soon, as the bursa will develop into a chronic niggling problem if you do. When you have allowed your shoulder enough rest for the inflammation to die down, you should do a programme of mobilizing and strengthening exercises for your shoulder for about a week or two, starting with easy exercises, in small quantities, and gradually increasing the amount you do. Once you can do the functional exercises without pain, you are safe to re-start your sport.

If, however, you do develop a recurrent problem with shoulder bursitis, or if the condition is very severe to start with, your doctor may refer you to an orthopaedic specialist with a view to having the painful bursa removed surgically. After the operation, your surgeon will tell you when to start exercising your shoulder, and you will follow the recovery process involving gradually strengthening and loosening the joint.

Biceps Tendon Tear

The biceps tendon, which passes through the shoulder joint, and then joins the bulky biceps muscle at the front of the shoulder, can be strained, like the other tendons around the shoulder. However, a severe strain can tear it completely, causing particular problems in the shoulder. This injury can happen when a strong contraction of the biceps is blocked, for instance if you are trying to make a hard throw, and an opponent pulls your arm suddenly backwards. Or it may happen when excessive loads create too much pressure in the muscle, for instance when a gymnast holds the crucifix position, holding his body-weight through the isometric holding power of his shoulder muscles.

What you feel is a sudden snap in the tendon, which may be very painful as it happens, or which may cause pain only afterwards. You see the bulky biceps muscle bunch up, leaving a noticeable gap between the muscle and the shoulder. You may also see some bruising and swelling over the front of the shoulder.

First-aid consists of ice applications, and a sling for support if the shoulder is very painful. As soon as possible, you should refer to the local casualty department, or your doctor. You may be referred to an orthopaedic specialist, with a view to having surgery to mend the broken tendon, and re-attach it to the bone, or stitch its two ends together, depending on the exact way in which it has torn. The specialist may decide to mend the tendon, but to allow the injury to heal naturally. Good functional recovery will be regained in the shoulder, although the tendon will not heal to its original state, and there may always be a slight weakness in the biceps muscle function.

Whether you have surgery or not, recovery consists of following a graduated programme of exercises to regain strength and flexibility in the shoulder. Your specialist will advise you on exactly when to start exercising the shoulder, and what exercises you should do. Generally, you start with gentle passive stretching for the front of the shoulder, avoiding causing any increasing pain. Strengthening starts with the isometric exercises and any of the dynamic strengthening exercises which you can do without pain. As with the simple shoulder strain, you progress gradually with the amount of movement and strengthening work you do, until you are fit to start with functional strengthening work, which leads up to re-starting sport. You should recover sufficiently to be able to do most normal and sporting activities without problems. However, you may have to accept that your shoulder might not regain enough power for highly demanding exercises, like the gymnast's crucifix.

Shoulder Dislocation

Dislocation of a joint means that one bone comes out of its retaining structures, causing pain, deformity and disability. At the shoulder, the top of the arm-bone springs out of its 'socket' of soft-tissue ligaments and its capsule. The shoulder is particularly vulnerable to this injury, because it is such a loose, mobile joint, and because in many sports it is subjected to violent wrenching strains. The only part of the shoulder that is protected by a bony structure is he top, which is covered by the arch formed between the collar-bone and the top ridge of the shoulder-blade. The top of the arm-bone may be pushed out forwards, downwards, or backwards. When it is wrenched out violently, the rounded head of he bone tears through the joint capsule and its ligaments, and through the surrounding muscles or tendons. If this happens, but the bone slips back into place immediately, the injury is called a subluxation.

This type of injury can occur if you fall on your hand at an angle from a height. When your arm is outstretched, your shoulder can easily be wrecked out of joint by an opponent's tackle in rugby, judo or wrestling. In swimmers, the injury may happened under relatively minor pressure, because the shoulder muscles over one side of the joint have the front of the shoulder is relatively weak, so the head of the arm-bone may slide forwards, while the opposite subluxation may happen to crawl swimmers.

Treatment

Then the injury happens violently, you should apply ice over your shoulder and support your arm in a comfortable position in a sling. You should not try to manipulate the joint back into place, but you should go to your doctor or casualty department for treatment.

If the injury has happened to you frequently, your doctor will probably refer you to an orthopaedic specialist. Surgery may be needed to restore stability in your shoulder.

After a shoulder operation, or after the initial phase of pain and disability, you must strengthen the shoulder specifically, before attempting your sport again. Start with the isometric exercises, and he simpler dynamic exercises, avoiding any which cause pain. Try to do two half-hour sessions a day, and do a few isometric exercises every hour during your normal activities. Once the shoulder is stronger, you can start doing the stretching and mobilizing exercises. You should only resume your sport when you have regained full power and mobility in your shoulder, and your specialist declares you fit.

You must maintain a daily routine of shoulder strengthening exercises, as this injury is very likely to keep happening. You may have to accept that you will be unable to continue high-risk sports like rugby, if the injury does recur, as even surgical repair is unlikely to make the joint strong enough against violent wrenching, although it normally given enough stability for sports like swimming.

Shoulder Exercises

Mobilizing Exercises

(i) Draw a straight line on the floor, fifteen centimetres away from a wall, and parallel to it. Stand with your toes against the line, facing the wall. Reach up as high as you can, to touch your fingers to the wall. Hold a pencil so that you can mark the wall, showing how high you can reach with each hand. Practise reaching up the wall from the same position each day, trying to reach further up each time with your injured arm.

(ii) Hold a towel or cord in both hands in front of you; swing your arms back over your head, keeping the towel taut, then swing back, ten times., Start with a long towel, and gradually shorten your grip.

(iii) Lying on your back with your hands clasped together, elbows straight, swing your arms upwards above your head, starting with twenty rhythmical swings forwards and back, and building up to fifty.

(iv) Standing with your legs apart, keeping your elbows straight, swing your arms forward and back to clap your hands in front of your chest and behind your back. Start with twenty free swinging movements, and build up to fifty.

(v) Holding a towel or cord behind your back, with one hand holding one end behind your head, and the lower end held in your other hand behind your back, pull at each end in turn to pull the towel up and down your back. Change hands to reverse the positions. Start with twenty quick movements, increasing to fifty. Use a fairly long towel at first, and gradually try to shorten your grip, to increase your shoulder movement.

(vi) With a weight in each hand, swing your arms easily forwards and backwards; then sideways and across your body; and finally round, describing large circles in the air. Start with twenty swings in each direction, building up to fifty.

(vii) Lying on your back with a bar held between your hands, and a weight strapped to the centre of the bar; swing the bar back over your head, rhythmically trying to swing your arms back a little further with each movement. Start with twenty swinging movements, and build up to fifty.

Dynamic Strengthening Exercises

(i) Wheelbarrow. With a partner holding your feet in the air, walk forwards, backwards and sideways on your hands. Without a partner, you can rest your feet up on a solid surface, and simply move around on your hands as far as you can, while keeping your feet on the support. Start with ten seconds of movement, building up to three minutes.

(ii) Using a light racket or bat, push a ball along the ground against a wall, in quick succession, gradually increasing your distance from the wall.

(iii) Press-ups. Start by kneeling on your hands and knees, then bend and straighten your elbows to do the press-ups. As soon as you are strong enough, do the full press-up, with your legs straight. Start with three, and build up to thirty.

(iv) Throw and catch a light ball with both hands, then one at a time, trying to increase the height of your throws gradually.

(v) Chins. Hanging from a bar, pull yourself up to touch your chin to the bar, the let your arms straighten fully before repeating the movement. Start with three, building up to three sets of ten.

(vi) Throw and catch a tennis-ball against a wall, overarm, underarm and sidearm. You should gradually increase your distance from the wall, so that you have to throw harder.

(vii) Backward Press-ups. With your legs straight out in front of you, and your hips off the floor, so that you are leaning back on your hands, bend and straighten your elbows. Start with three, build to three sets of ten.

(viii) Crab-walking. Resting your weight backwards on your feet and hands, 'walks' forwards, backwards and sideways. Start with fifteen seconds, and build up to three minutes.

(ix) Hanging from a bar, pull yourself up to touch the back of your head gently to the bar. Start with three, build up to three sets of ten.

Isometric Strengthening Exercises

(i) With your injured arm held out sideways, at right angles to your body, and your elbow bent, so that your hand is up in the air, press your other hand against your palm, to block the movement as you try to press your hand downwards, as if trying to turn your arm at the shoulder, and not allowing your elbow to change its position. Hold to five, then relax.

(ii) With your injured arm by your side, place your other hand on the back of your arm, just above the elbow. Blocking the movement with your hand, press your arm backwards for a count of five, then relax.

(iii) With your arm held up by your head, and the elbow bent over your head, press your other hand against your palm, to resist the forward turning movement. Hold to five, then relax.

(iv) Keeping your injured arm straight by your side, while your are sitting or standing, place your other hand just above the outside of your elbow. Using this hand to block any movement, press your injured arm outwards, away from your side to increase the muscle tension at your shoulder. Hold the contraction for a count of five, then relax completely.

(v) With your injured arm by your side, place your other hand on the front of your arm, just above your elbow. Blocking the movement with your hand, press your arm forwards for a count of five, then relax.

(vi) Repeat (ii), (iv) and (v) with your arm held out sideways at an angle of ninety degrees to your body.

(vii) With your arm held sideways, elbow bent, place your other hand to resist the backward turning movement by pressing against the back of your hand. Hold to five, then relax.

(viii) With your arm at your side, and the elbow bent, place your other hand against the back of your hand,. Keeping your elbow at your side, try to press your hand outwards, against the resistance of the other hand. Hold the contraction for a count of five, the relax completely.

(ix) With your injured arm by your side, and your elbow bent to a right angle, place your other hand against the palm of the hand on your injured arm. Blocking the movement with your other hand, press the palm of your hand inwards, without letting your elbow move, as though you were trying to take your forearm across your stomach. Hold the contraction for a count of five, then relax completely.

Strengthening Exercises

(i) Sitting or standing, lift both arms straight forward above your head, keeping your arms close to your head, slowly lower. Build up to three sets of ten, then add in weights.

(ii) Shoulder pull. Using a weight machine or pull system, using gradually increasing weights, pull the bar downwards, hold for a count of three, then slowly control the return movement. Build up to three sets of ten.

(iii) Shoulder press. With a weighted bar held behind your neck on your shoulders, straighten your arms upwards in the air, hold for a count of three, then slowly lower. Start with light weights, building up to three sets of ten, then gradually increase the weights.

(iv) Lying on your back, with your injured arm held across your body so that your hand rests on he opposite hip, lift your arm straight upwards and slightly sideways, turning it so that the palm of your hand faces towards your head, so that your arm stretches back to lie beside your head. Slowly lower. Build up to three sets of ten, then add in weights.

(v) Sitting on standing, raise both arms straight out sideways, hold for a count of three, then slowly lower. Start with three sets of five lifts, build up to three sets of ten, then do the exercise with light weights in your hands, gradually increasing the weights.

(vi) Dips. On a weights machine, or sitting between two chairs or parallel bars, lift yourself up by pushing on your hands; or push the machine handles downwards; hold for a count of three, then slowly return to the starting position. Build up to three sets of ten.

(vii) Sitting or standing, lift up both arms, bending your elbows to touch the palms of your hands on the back of your head, then lower your arms, bending them so that you touch your lower back with the backs of your hands. Start with twenty movements in quick succession, then add in weights.

(viii) Sit or stand with your arms held straight out sideways; take your arms straight forwards, to touch your hands, the stretch them out sideways again. Build up to three sets of the, then add in weights.

(ix) Lying on your back, at the edge of a couch or bed, so that your arm lies over the side, keeping your elbow straight, take your arm up and across your body, to cross the other shoulder. Start the movement with your palm facing upwards, and turn your arm as you lift it, so that your palm faces downward at the end of the movement. Slowly lower back. Build up to three sets of ten, then add in weights.

(x) Sitting on standing, lift both arms straight forward, hold for a count of three, then slowly lower. Build up to three sets of ten, then add in weights.

Stretching Exercises

(i) With your arm bent over your head, pull your wrist sideways with your other hand. As you pull you your arm over your head, bend sideways in the same direction, until you feel the stretch across the underside of your shoulder. Hold to ten, then relax.

(ii) Lying under a low bar, just further than an arm's length from the floor, take your weight on your hands by grasping the bar, keeping your body stretched straight out in front of you. Relax your shoulder completely, so that you feel the stretch over your upper trunk and the back of your shoulder-joints. Hold the position for as long as you are comfortable.

(iii) Hold a lightly weighted bar up above your head, with your elbows straight and your hands a shoulder's width apart. Stretch your arms backwards, hold for ten, then relax completely.

(iv) Triceps. Lift your arm straight up in the air, then bend your elbow so that your hand is behind your head. With your other hand, pull your elbow towards your head, until you feel the stretch at the back of your arm. Hold this position for a count of ten, then relax.

(v) Keeping your elbows straight, clasp your hands together above your head. Stretch your arms backwards, hold for a count of ten, then relax.

(vi) Hang from a bar by your hands, and let your shoulders relax completely. Hold the position for as long as you are comfortable, the step down.

(vii) With your arm bent over your head, pull your wrist sideways with your other hand. As you pull your arm over your head, bend sideways in the same direction, until you feel the stretch across the underside of your shoulder. Hold to ten, then relax.

Complications

Chronic stiffness

If you do not make a complete recovery from a shoulder injury, but your re-start your sport too soon, or if you suffer repeated injuries to your shoulder, the joint may get gradually stiffer, because you are no longer able to use it fully. You may not notice this happening, until you reach the stage when you cannot lift your arm above your head. As the joint stiffens, it is also weakened. As soon as you notice this happening, you must start doing mobilizing exercises, and isometric ad simple dynamic strengthening exercises. You may have to work through pain in your shoulder, but it is essential to reverse the process of progressive stiffness ad weakness. You should also refer to your doctor for a check, just in case there is some underlying medical reason for the stiffness, apart from simple loss of function.

Acromio-Clavicular Joint Strain

After a shoulder injury, you may find that you have localized pain over the top of the shoulder, and soreness if you carry a heavy weight in your hand. This may mean that when you injured your shoulder, you also injured the joint between your collar-bone and the ridge on your shoulder-blade. The damage done may vary from a strain of the ligaments binding the joint, to a total tear of the ligaments, but the problem may not be evident until the pain in your shoulder has subsided. If the injury is severe, you may feel the separation between the two bones over the top of your shoulder. You must refer to your doctor, as the condition can last a long time, if it is to treated.

8

CARE AND PREVENTION OF FOOT AND ANKLE INJURIES

Abour 55% per cent to 90% of sports injuries involve the lower extremity, most commonly the knee, foot, and ankle. The majority of foot and ankle injuries are related to running, jumping, or cutting manoeuvres.

Acute foot and ankle injuries account for 10% of emergency department visits. Overuse injuries are also common, however, and most often are not seen in an emergency setting.

Overuse syndromes in the foot account for 50% of injuries. The highest incidence in the series reported by Garrick and Requa occurred in volleyball; running and tennis, racquetball, and gymnastics has the next highest incidence rates. Sprains do occur in the foot, but they account for less than 7% of foot injuries.

Knowledge of the anatomy and clinical data are essential requirements for optimal imaging of the foot and ankle. Therefore, these aspects of foot and ankle injuries are emphasized along with specific imaging techniques.

Anatomy

Basic osseous and soft tissue anatomy is discussed here.

Osseous and Ligamentous Anatomy of the Ankle

The ankle is formed by three bones: The tibia, and fibula, and the talus. The tibia is the second longest bone in the skeleton. It is expanded proximally and distally. The body of the tibia has three surfaces: anterior, medial, and posterior. The anterior surface ends in the medial mellifluous. The medial margin is subcutaneous. The interosseous membrane attaches to the lateral margin.

The anterior surface of the tibia is smooth except at the anteroinferior margin, where it is more irregular at the site for attachment of the anterior ankle capsule. The posterior tibia has grooves for the flexor hallucis longus and flexor digitorum longus and tibialis posterior tendons. The lateral surface articulates with the fibula. This articular surface is bounded anteriorly and posteriorly by ridges for insertion of the anterior and posterior distil tibiofibular ligaments. The strong medial extension articulates with the talus and forms the medial portion of the ankle mortise.

The fibula is this and flat and does not have a direct weightbearing surface. The lateral malleolus is the expanded distal portion of the fibula. The fibula is irregular along its medial margin at the point of attachment for the interosseous ligament. Hyaline carilage covers the articular surface on the inferomedial aspect. There are irregular areas anteriorly and posteriorly for insertions of the tibiofibular ligament. The fibula is more posterior than the medical malleolus, and its distal extent is below the level of the medical malleolar tip. Thus an angle of about 8° is formed by a line drawn from the tips of the malleoli. The posterior position of the lateral malleolus results in an angle of 20° between the malleoli in the axial plane. For this reason the mortise view of the ankle is taken with the foot internally rotated approximately 20°.

The hyaline cartilage trochlear surface of the talus is usually 2 to 3 mm wider anteriorly than posteriorly. It articulares with the weight-bearing surface of the tibia and the medial and lateral malleoli. Thus the ankle mortise is formed by the tibial and fibular components of the ankle, which roofs the talus. The tibial portion of the mortise is termed the plafond. Forces on the talus that result in position changes of this structure in the mortise are responsible for many osseous and/or ligamentous ankle injuries.

The deltiod ligament provides medial stability. This ligament is strong, triangular-shaped group of fibres with its apex at the medial maleolus. The ligament fans out as it progresses inferiorly and divides into superficial and deep fibres. The superficial fibres insert in the navicular tuberosity. Progressing posteriorly, the remaining superficial fibres insert in the sustentaculum tali and the talus. The deep fibres attach to the medial surface of the talus. The deltoid ligament prevents excessive abduction and eversion of the ankle and subtalar joints. In addition, eversion, pronation, and anterior displacement of the talus are restricted.

Foot Anatomy

For purposes of discussion, the foot can be divided into three segments: the hindfoot, midfoot, and forefoot. Three longitudinal columns have also been described. The medial column consists of the calcaneus, talus, navicular, medial and intermediate cuneiforms, and first and second metatarsals and phalanges. The middle column consists of the lateral cuneiform and the third metatarsal and phalanx. The lateral column is made up of the hindfoot and the fourth and fifth metatarsals with their phalanges. All articulations are synovial joints supported by strong plantar and weaker dorsal ligaments.

Hindfoot

The hindfoot includes the talus and calcaneus. The

talus is the second largest of the tarsal bones and articulates with the tibia, medial and lateral malleoli, and calcaneus inferiorly. The talar head artisculates with the navicular.

Superiorly the trochlea articulates with the tibia and malleoli. It is covered with hyaline cartilage and makes up the upper portion of the body of the talus. There are three articular facets on the inferior surface of the talus. The anterior and posterior facets articulate with similarly named calcaneal articular facet. The middle facet articulates with the sustentaculum tali. The talar sulus lies between the middle and anterior facets. The structure with its calcaneal counterpart forms the tarsal sinu, which contains the interosseous talocalcaneal ligament. The head of the talus articulates with the navicular.

Several osseous growths have been described on the talus. These are usually of no clinical significance. A normal ridge is present distal to the trochlear surface on the dorsolateral aspect of the talus. This can be seen on the lateral view of the ankle and should not be confused with pathology. This ridge is the site of attachment of the dorsal talonavicular ligament and anterior tibviotalar joint capsule. Therefore, hypertrophy can occur in patients engaged in activities that require extremes of planter flexion. The posterior aspect of the talus contains an oblique groove for the flexor hallucis longus tendon.

The calcaneus, which is the largest tarsal bone, contains three superior articular facets. The middle, most medial facet is on the sustentaculum tali. The calcaneal sulcus lies between the middle and anterior facets and forms the floor of the tarsal canal. This canal has an oblique course and measures 10 to 15 mm is height, 3 to 5 mm in width, and 15 to 20 mm in length. The distal or plantar surface of the calcaneus contains two grooves. The lateral groove. The lateral groove is for the peroneus longus tendon. More medially, the flexor hallucis longus runs in the groove beneath the sustentaculum tali.

Midfoot

The remaining tarsal bones make up the midfoot. These include the cubiod, the navicular, and three cuneiforms.

The cuboid articulates with the calcaneus proximally and with the fourth and fifth metatarsals distally. Dorsally the cuboid is roughened at the points of ligament attachment. On the planter surface the cuboid contains a groove for the peroneus longus tendon. The medial cuboid surface contains a facet font articulation with the lateral cuneiform.

The navicular is on the medial side of the foot anterior to the talus. It articulates proximally with the talus, anteriorly with the cuneiforms, and occasionally laterally with the cuboid.

The spring ligament is contiguous with the deltoid ligament of the ankle. It extends from the calcaneus to the navicular tuberosity. The cubonavicular ligament runs dorsally from the cuboid to the navicular. Proximally the bifurcate ligament originates on the anterosuperior calcaneus and sends medial fibres to the lateral navicular and lateral fibres to the cuboid. The calcaneonavicular ligament is on the plantar aspect of the capsule.

There are three cuneiform bones located distal to the navicular and medial to the cuboid. The medial cuneiform is the largest and articulates with the navicular proximally, the intermediate cuneiform laterally, and the first and second metatarsal distally.

The intermediate cuneiform is the smallest cuneiform and lies between the medial and lateral cuneiforms. It articulates with the latter bones, the navicular, and the second metatarsal. The lateral cuneiform lies between the intermediate cuneiform and the cuboid, articulating with both. It also articulates with the navicular and the second through fourth metatarsals.

The five metatarsals articulate proximally with the tarsal bones described above, and each, except the first, typically has three phalanges distally. The metatarsals have a similar configuration except that the first is broader from the proximal articular surface distally to its head. The fifth metatarsal has a broad base compared to the second through fourth metatarsals.

Arches of the Foot

There are three arches in the foot: one transverse and two longitudinal. The lateral longitudinal arch is formed by the calcanesus, cuboid, and fourth and fifth metatarsals. In a patient with normal gait, this arch normally receives the weight of the body before the medial longitudinal arch. The peroneus longus tendon runs through the midpoint of this arch. The medial longitudinal arch is formed by the calcaneus, talus, navicular, cuneiforms, and first through third metatarsals. The vertical height of the medial arch is greater than that of the lateral arch. The apex of the arch is more posterior, being located at the calcaneotalonavicular junction. The posterior tibial tendon inserts on the navicular and sends plantar fibres below the arch, adding additional support.

The transverse arch is completed when the feet are adjacent, so that the two medial longitudinal arches are approximated. Thus the bases of the metatarsals and midtarsal bones form the arch with support from the peroneus longus and posterior tibial tendons.

Normal Variants

There are many anatomical variants that can mimic more serious pathologic conditions. These changes are most common in the metaphyseal and epihyseal areas adjacent to the growth plates. Occassionally small ossification centres are evident adjacent to he growth plates, simulating fractures. Ossicles are also commonly noted near the medial and lateral malleoli. These frequently cause confusion in diagnosing patients with recent injury. They occur medially in 17% to 14% of girls and up to 47% of boys. Most are bilateral, and they are commonly seen from 6 to 12 years. Normal variants are also common in the tarsal bones.

The secondary ossification centre of the talus is located posteriorly. It appears at 8 to 11 years of age and normally fuses at 16 to 20 years of age. This somewhat controversial ossification centre is the posterior part of the talar tubercle and is located lateral to the flexor hallucis longus tendon. If this centre does not fuse to the talus, it is called the so trigonum tarsi and is frequently mistaken for a fracture. In forced plantar the ossicle can separate, or fracture can occur in the fused centre.

Another common finding is the accessory navicular, or as tibial externum. This lies in the posterior tibial tendon just proximal to the medial margin of the navicular. This ossicle may affect tendon function, especially during puberty when growth is accelerated. Resection may be required to relieve the painful symptoms. The os supranaviculatre is located at the proximal dorsal margin of the navicular distal to the joint space. This is more distal than the os supratalare, which would be proximal to the talonavicular joint. The most frequently noted ossicles in the foot are summarized in.

Soft Tissue Anatomy

The muscles of the calf are divided into anterior, posterior, and lateral compartments. Because of their action on the foot and ankle, a brief review of anatomy and function is in indicated.

The muscles of the deep posterior compartment also act on the foot and ankle except for the populates, which serves as a flexor of the knee. The flexor hallucis longus serves as a flexor of the great toe, and the flexor digitorum longus assists in plantar flexing the foot and serves as a flexor of the lateral four toes. The tibialis posterior is the deepest muscle of the posterior compartment. Its tendon passes anterior to the flexor digitorum under the flexor retinaculum to insert on the navicular and tarsal bones. This muscle aids in adduction, inversion, and plantar flexion. Neurovascular supply to the posterior muscles is via the tibial nerve and posterior tibial artery.

The personas longus and brevis are the muscles of the lateral compartment. The tendons enter a common sheath above the ankle and pass posterior to the lateral malleolus and deep to the peroneal retinacula. On the tateral surface of the foot the peroneus brevis inserts on the lateral surface of the foot the peroneus brevis inserts on the fifth metatarsal base. The peroneus longus passes under the foot to insert on the medial cuneiform and first metatarsal base. Both muscles assist in eversion and plantar flexion of the foot.

The anterior compartment comprises the extensor digitorum longus, peroneus tertius, extensor hallucis longus, and tibialis anterior. The extensor digitorum longus aids in dorsiflextion of the foot and lateral four toes. The extensor hallucis longus serves mainly for dorsiflextion of the great toe. The tibialis anterior inserts at the midfoot and aids in dorsiflexion and inversion of the foot. Neurovascular supply to the anterior and lateral compartments is via the peroneal nerve and anterior tibial and peroneal arteries.

The musculature of the foot is complex. A complete discussion of origins and insertions is beyond the scope of this text. Certain functional aspects will be discussed, but the reader is referred to other texts of a more in-depth discussion. The muscles of the foot are divided into four layers. The superficial muscles include the abductor hallucis, flexor digitorum brevis and abductor digit minimi. The former is a weak abductor of the great toe and is supplied by the medial plantar artery and nerve. The centrally located flexor digitorum brevis has the same neurovascular supply. It serves as a flexor of the lateral four toes. The abductor digit minimi is a flexor and abductor of the fifth toe.

The second layer of muscles includes the quadratus plantae, lumbrical muscles, and tendons of the flexor hallucis longus and flexor digitiorum longus. These muscles assist in flexion of the toes. Neurovascular supply is via both medial and lateral plantar artery and nerve branches.

The third layer includes the flexor hallucis brevis, adductor hallucis, and flcxor digiti minimi brevis. The flexor hallucis aids in flexion of the great toe, and the adductor hallucis serves as an adductor of the great toe. The flexor digiti minimi flexes the small toe.

The fourth and deepest muscle layer includes the three painter and four dorsal interosseous muscles. The dorsal interossei act as abductors and the plantar interossei as adductors of the foot.

The extensor digitorum brevis is the dorsal muscle of the foot. The muscle is a corsiflexor of the great toe and second through fourth toes.

Common Terms

Terms used to describe the movements in the foot and ankle are often misused. This results in some confusion when descriptive terms such as supination, eversion, pronation, and the like are used. Definitions of these commonly used terms are listed below as they apply during physiologic motion of the foot and ankle.

- Plantar flexion: The hinge motion at the tibiolalar joint allows the foot to plantar flex. Several other motions and position changes occur with plantar flexion. During plantar flexion the gastrocnemius muscle pulls the calcaneus upward, which shifts the calcaneus into a slight varus position. The head of the talus turns in and downward during plantar flexion, which causes the foot to move inward.
- Dorsiflexion: The hinge motion of the ankle allows the foot to be elevated or dorsiflexed. The gastrocnemius muscle is relaxed, and the heel shifts into a valgus position. The talus turns upward and outward, so that the foot also furns outward during dorsiflexion.
- Inversion: During inversion the sole of the foot is turned inward. In the European literature the terms supination and adduction are often used interchangeably with inversion. The foot tends to dorsiflex slightly during inversion.
- Eversion: During eversion the sole of the foot is turned outward. The terms pronation and abduction have been used interchangeably with eversion. The foot tends to plantar flex slightly during eversion.
- Adduction: By definition, adduction means movement of a part toward the axis or midline. The

term is most frequently used to describe forces acting on the foot or ankle. Inversion has been equated with adduction in the literature. The term adduction is preferred when describing forces applied to the foot and ankle.

- Abduction: This term indicates motion of a given part away from the midline. Again, terms such as eversion have been used interchangeably with abduction; abduction is preferred when describing forces moving the foot or ankle outward.
- Supination and pronation: Supination and pronation are commonly used for describing the rotation that occurs at the wrist. Technically the foot is pronated when the sole is flat. Pronation can occur to a minimal degree with the forefoot abducted and dorsiflexed. Limited supination is possible. Typically the literature has used the terms pronation and eversion, and supination and inversion, interchangeably. The terms supination and pronation should be reserved for the upper extremity. Eversion and inversion are less confusing when describing foot and ankle position.
- External rotation: The term is typically used to define outward rotation of the foot in relation to the longitudinal axis of the leg. With many athletic injuries the leg actually rotates medially with the foot fixed. Therefore, the foot then is actually rotated in an outward position compared to the leg.
- Varus: Varus indicates rotation, bending, or positioning inward or toward the midline axis. The term should be used to describe position, not motion.
- Valgus: Valgus is used to denote rotation, bending, or positioning away from the axis of the midline.

Like varus, the term valgus denotes position.

Soft Tissue Trauma

Injuries affecting the soft tissues of the foot and ankle are common. Cass and Morrey reported and incidence of about 500 ankle sprains per year. Sprains in the foot occur less frequently. Many injuries can be treated conservatively with satisfactory results. Proper imaging evaluation, however, is needed to determine the extent of injury so that chronic instability and function loss can be avoided.

Ankle Ligament Injuries

Certain aspects of ankle anatomy bear repeating, however, to provide a complete discussion of ligamentous trauma.

The distal tibia and fibula are supported in their anatomic relationship by the distal anterior and posterior tibiofibular ligaments and the interosseous membrance Other ligament structures maintain the ankle joint. Medially, the deltiod ligament is triangular and broadens as it extends from the medial malleolus to its talar and calcaneal insertions. The deltoid ligament is composed of an anterior and posterior superficial ligament and an intermediate deep or tibiotalar ligament. The latter ligament is essentially a triangular thickening with a medial capsule. There are three ligaments laterally. The anterior talofibular ligament extends from the anterior fibula to insert in the lateral talus just below the articular surface. With the ankle in a neutral position, this ligament is horizontally oriented and resists internal rotation. Recent studies also indicate that it is significant in resisting varus tilt, particularly with the ankle in plantar flexion. The posterior tibiofibular ligament extends from the posterior fibula to the posterior talus. The clacaneofibular ligament originates at the lateral malleolar tip and inserts on the calcaneus, restricting inversion. The calcaneofibular ligament supports both the ankle and the subtalar joints and is intimately associated with the peroneal tendon sheaths.

Diagnosis of ligament disruption usually requires special studies. Toutine ankle views are not effective in differentiating the types of ankle sprains. Secondary signs, however, are important in determining which additional techniques may be most useful. Patients with grade 1 sprains generally present with mild soft tissue swelling over the lateral malleolus. This can be identified on AP and mortise views. A bright light is frequently needed to evaluate the soft tissues. No fracture or effusion is evident on the lateral view. Grade 2 and 3 sprains have more significant selling that can be identified clinically and on both AP and lateral radiographs. This finding has little value, however. Attempts at correlating ligament injury with the degree of swelling seen radiographically have been unsuccessful. The presence of an effusion in the joint is somewhat useful in that is generally indicates that the capsule is intact. Effusions are best seen on the lateral view. Small avulsion fractures can also be seen on plain films. Measuring the tibiotalar joint to differentiate second- and third-degree sprains is not usually helpful. It the talus is shifted, however, resulting in asymmetry of the ankle mortise, a ligament injury is generally present.

Stress views are less accurate compared to arthrography or tenography. Sauser et al studied 55 patients with stress views and arthrography within 72 hours of injury. They noted that stress views were accurate if talar tilt increased by 10° or more but that the test was only positive in 38% of patients with positive arthrograms.

This decision should be based on clinical findings and whether surgery or treatment modifications will be made as judged from the degree of ligament injury. Surgical intervention is a more important consideration in professional athletes or young active individuals. Generally, assessment of the calcaneofibular ligament is most crucial because conservative treatment is most often used if only the anterior talofibular ligament is torn. Therefore, a stress tenogram is the technique of choice. Computed tomography and MRI are useful in evaluating the tendons around the ankle but, in our experience, are less effective in evaluating the capsule and ligaments.

Ligament injuries also occur in the foot. Gymnastics, long distance running, and aerobic activities are frequently implicated. Inversion injuries, which may mimic typical ankle sprains, may affect the bifurcate ligament, which extends between the calcaneus and cuboid. Other midtarsal ligaments are also stressed in gymnasts and dancers. Diagnosis of these conditions may be difficult clinically.

Cuboid subluxation may be particularly difficult to diagnose. The athlete typically presents with lateral midfoot pain and is unable to run, cut, or jump. Pain or point tenderness may be noted on plantar pressure over the cuboid.

Sinus tarsi syndrome is commonly associated with inversion injuries of the foot and ankle sprains. The talocalcaneal interosseous ligament carries the hidfoot nerve fibres, and even minor injury may cause significant pain. On physical examination there is point tenderness over the lateral aspect of the sinus tarsi.

Middle-aged joggers commonly develop subluxation of the metatarsophalangeal joint, specifically the second joint Patients present with metatarsal pain and often have claw toe deformities.

Imaging of ligament injuries of the foot is difficult. Routine radiographs, CT, or conventional tomography may be useful to identify subtle associated avulsion fractures. MRI is useful in specific situations. Diagnostic and therapeutic injections, however, are most useful in localizing the pain and confirming the clinical diagnosis. Fluorscopically monitored injections can be accomplished in all articulations. A mixture of bupivacaine and betamethasone is injected after confirming needle position with a small amount of contrast medium.

Tendon Injuries

Thirteen tendons cross the ankle. These tendons include the peroneus brevis and longus laterally; the Achilles tendon posteriorly; the tibialis posterior, flexor digitorum longus, and flexor hallucis longus medially; and the tibialis anterior, extensor hallucis longus, extensor digitiorum longus, and peroneus tertius anteriorly. All tendons are enclosed in sheaths with the exception of the Achilles tendon. Tendon injury may occur as an isolated event, in association with a fracture, or as a result of previous fracture with degenerative joint disease. Tendons may also rupture in patients on steroid therapy or with chronic inflammatory diseases.

Peroneal Tendons

The peroneal muscles assist in pronation and eversion of the foot. The peroneus brevis tendon is anterior to the peroneus longus as they pass posterior to the lateral malleoulus. In about 80% of patients there is a notch in the fibula that accommodates a portion of the peroneus brevis. In 20% of patients this notch is shallow or absent, which may lead to recurrent subluxation. Thetendons also through the superior and inferior peroneal retinacula. It is between these two structures that they are immediately adjacent to the calcaneofibular ligament. The peroneal tendons share a common sheath to the inferior margin of the superior peroneal retinaculum. At this point the sheath of the peroneus longus separates from that of the peroneus brevis. The peroneus longus progresses inferior to the peroneal tubercle of the calcaneus to the plantar aspect of the foot, where it inserts in the base of the first metatarsal and medial cuneiform. The peroneus brevis passes inferiorly, inserting on the base of the fifth metatarsal. Evaluation of the tendons and normal osseous sulci is easily accomplished with MRI or CT.

Dislocation. Diagnosis of peroneal tendon injury first requires that the problem be considered. Many patients present with a sprained ankle or repeated giving-way, and dislocation of the peroneal tendons is not considered. The mechanism of injury is not clear, but dislocation is probably due to an inversion-dorsiflexion or abduction-dorsiflexion injury. Patients present with pain and swelling over the posterosuperior aspect of the lateral malleolus.

Swelling may make actual palpation of the tendon difficult, and pain with motion can limit the detection of subluxation on physical examination. Routine radiographs will demonstrate soft tissue swelling laterally, but the distribution is not characteristic or different from that of an inversion sprain. A characteristic longitudinal flake fracture along the distal fibular metaphysis is useful when present. This is best seen on the internal oblique view. Murr reported this finding in 15% to 50% of peroneal tendon dislocations. Usually other imaging procedures are more useful. CT, MRI, or tenography should be considered to confirm the diagnosis. CT provides excellent bone detail and is useful in assessing the peroneal notch in the fibula. The tendons are less well demonstrated with CT than with MRI. Subtle tears or complete disruptions are more easily seen on MRI, where the tendons are normally of low signal intensity compared to the high intensity seen in the tendon that has torn. These nonivasive techniques do have disadvantages. For example, if the tendons have returned to normal position or are only slightly displaced, fluoroscopic observation after tenography may be more useful in demonstrating subluxation. This may also be possible to demonstrate with new fast-scan MR techniques.

Rupture of the peroneal tendon. Rupture of the peroneal tendons is not common. The lesion may be overlooked as a cause of ankle instability, however, and therefore the true incidence is not known. Patients may present acutely with an ankle sprain or have symptoms of chronic instability. Cavovarus foot and compartment syndromes have also been reported with peroneal tendon rupture. When the tendons are torn, the patient will be unable effectively to evert the foot.

Routine radiographs are usually not useful. Displacement of the os peroneum, however, may indicate peroneal rupture. Tenography may demonstrate the site of the tear, but because this technique outlines the tendon and does not provide direct assessment it is less useful than MRI. Both CT and MRI have been described as useful techniques for evaluating the peroneal tendons. MRI has superior soft tissue contrast and can define incomplete, complete, and chronic inflammatory changes in both the tendon and the sheath. If a complete tear is present, the tendon ends can be defined as well as the absence of the tendon in its sheath in the torn region. If a partial tear has occurred there will be increased signal intensity in the tendon due to blood and fluid. These findings are most easily demonstrated on T2-weighted or gradient-echo T2* sequences. The contrast of the blood and fluid compared to the normally low-intensity tendon is most striking with these sequences. In patients with old tears the tendon will look thickened with areas of intermediate intensity, and there is often fluid in the tendon sheath. The latter is not seen in normal patients.

Achilles Tendon

The Achilles tendon is the largest and strongest tendon in the foot and ankle. The tendon originates where the gastrocnemius and soleus tendons join and inserts on the posterior calcaneus. In its axial presentation the tendon thickens distally, becoming elliptical with concave anterior and convex posterior surfaces. Approximately 2 to 6 cm above its calcaneal insertion, the fibres in the tendon cross. The posterior fibres course medial to lateral, and the anterior fibres lateral to medial, before inserting in the calcaneus. Most tendon tears occur just above this, perhaps partially because of the reduced blood supply in this region. The Achilles tendon does not have a true tendon sheath.

Acute and chronic inflammation of the Achilles tendon is common in runners. Up to 11% or runners develop Achilles tendinitis. Inflammation is usually due to errors in training. The injury is also common in request sports and most commonly occurs in 30- to 50-year-old men.

The Achilles tendon, although strong, is commonly torn. Fifty-nine percent of ruptures are related to sports injuries. Ruptures are usually the result of indirect trauma. The injury can occur during athletic activity at any age. It usually occurs in strenuous activities with frequent plantar flexion during raising up on the toes or with pushing off or jumping with the knee extended. Falling or landing on the forefoot, which leads to abrupt dorsiflexion of the foot, can also lead to Achilles rupture. Certain systemic and local conditions predispose to tendon disruption. Gout, systemic lupus erythematosus, rheumatoid arthritis, hyperparathyroidism, chronic renal failure, steroids, and diabetes have all been implicated.

In addition to ruptures, Achilles tendinitis is one of the most common overuse syndromes. Because there is no tendon sheath, the peritenon becomes inflamed. Inflammation is frequently related to footwear and a pronated heel and is seen in runners who use hilly terrain.

Imaging of Achilles tendon pathology can be accomplished with several modalities. Routine radiographs are usually nonspecific. Newmark et al, however, described fracture of a calcaneal osteophyte in association with Achilles tendon avulsion. Low-kilovoltage radiography and Xerox techniques may demonstrate swelling, thickening of the tendon, and irregularity of the pre-Achilles fat or Kager's triangle. These findings are best seen on the lateral view. Ultrasound can also be effective in elucidating the architecture of the tendon. This requires experience on the part of the examiner and interpreter. Ultrasound images can be difficult to interpret by those who do not routinely use the technique.

CT and MRI, although more expensive than the techniques mentioned above, provide more information about the tendon and surrounding structures. MRI is particularly useful because of its superior soft tissue contrast and ability to image in the axial, sagittal, coronal, and off-axis oblique planes. At the Mayo clinic, we find MRI to be useful in detecting complete, incomplete and old Achilles injuries as well as in evaluating bursitis and other causes of Achilles tendon pathology. The extent of involvement can be assessed accurately with MRI. In addition, patients can be followed to determine whether healing is progressing normally or whether operative intervention is necessary.

Another uncommon problem may mimic and Achilles injury or soft tissue tumour. This situation is created by the presence of an accessory soleus muscle. It is not uncommon for a patients with this anomaly to experience pain after exercise. Either CT or MRI can easily diagnose the condition, but MRI can more easily distinguish the accessory soleus muscle from a soft tissue tumor or hematoma.

Medial Tendons

The posterior tibial, flexor digitorum longus, and flexor hallucis longus tendons make up the medial tendon group and are located anterior to posterior in the above order. The posterior tibial tendon with its tendon sheath passes just posterior to the medial malleolus and lateral to the flexor retinaculum and broadens at its insertion in the navicular tuberosity and base of the medial cuneiform. The flexor digitorum longus takes a similar course proximally, lying between the posterior tibial tendon and the posterior tibial artery. As it turns towards the plantar aspect of the foot, it passes superficially to the flexor hallucis longus before dividing into tendon slips that insert in the bases of the second to fifth distal phalanges. The flexor hallucis longus tendon is located more posteriorly and laterally. It passes through a fibroosseous tunnel beneath the sustentaculum tali and along the medial plantar aspect of the foot to insert in the base of the distal phalanx of the great toe.

Acute rupture of the deltoid ligament is not common. Similarly, the posterior tibial, flexor digitorum longus, and flexor hallucis longus tendons are rarely torn after acute trauma. Zezwart and Davidson have reported posterior tibial tendon rupture in association with bimalleolar fracture.

The posterior tibial tendon is the most commonly injured of the three medial tendons. Injury typically occurs during the pronation phase in running or with rapid changes in direction in basketball, soccer, football, and tennis. Patients present with pain, local tenderness, and swelling, and physical examination may reveal a nonpalpable tendon. Rupture of the posterior tibial tendon can lead to progressive flatfoot deformity, inability to raise up on the toes, and weakness on inversion of the foot.

Routine radiography is usually of little value in patients with medial tendon injuries. Acute traumatic rupture of the posterior tibial tendon has been described in association with medial malleolar fractures. The fracture is a mirror image of the flake fracture seen with peroneal tendon dislocation. It occurs longitudinally along the distal medial tibial metaphysis. Posterior tibial tendon rupture may present with an increased tolocalcaneal angle on the AP and lateral view. These findings, along with soft tissue swelling, are the only plain film findings that might suggest the diagnosis. In patients with chronic disease and inflammation, the stress tenogram may show changes in the posterior tibial or adjacent tendon sheaths. The structure of the tendon is better demonstrated with CT or MRI, however. In our experience MRI has been most useful in assessing the nature and degree of posterior tibial tendon pathology.

Rupture of the flexor digitorum and flexor hallucis longus tendons occurs less frequently but can present with similar clinical findings. Garth reported rupture of the flexor hallucis longus in ballet dancers and soccer players. Patients presented with swelling, tenderness, and crepitation near the sustentaculum tali. Symptoms were increased with flexion and extension of the great toe.

Tenography of the flexor hallucis longus is tedious because of the difficulty in localizing the tendon with the needle tip. Therefore, MRI or CI is more useful.

Anterior Tendons

Anteriorly the anterior tibial, extensor hallucis longus, and extensor digitorum longus tendons are all enclosed in tendon sheaths. Acute tears are unusual, but in patients with previous fractures, degenerative arthritis, or other predisposing factors tendon rupture can occur. Chronic inflammation or more significant involvement of the anterior tibial tendon is not uncommon in runners. Rupture of the anterior tibial tendon usually occurs as it exits the superior retinaculum. The distal segment retracts and can be palpated between the superior and inferior retinacula. Clinically there is pain and swelling over the ankle anteriorly. There may also be decreased dorsiflextion of the foot on physical examination.

Radiographically patients will demonstrate minimal to prominent soft tissue swelling anteriorly. This is most easily identified on the lateral and oblique views.

Hindfoot Pain

Hindfoot and/or heel pain is common in athletes. For purposes of discussion, it is useful to consider four different areas plantar, posterior, lateral, and medial.

Plantar Pain

The most common problem resulting in plantar pain is fasciitis. The condition is noted in 7% of runners. In the acute phase there is more focal pain at the medial calcaneal attachment, but with prolonged symptoms the pain and area of tenderness on physical examination become more diffuse. The condition is more common with cavus foot or excessive pronation.

Routine radiography may demonstrate distortion of soft tissue planes or periostitis. These changes are most easily appreciated on the lateral view. Although radionuclide scans may be useful, MRI is most effective for differentiation of inflammation from ruptures of the plantar fascia.

Medial calcaneal nerve entrapment may also lead to plantar pain. The condition is most often noted in runners, and some investigators postulate the syndrome is caused by inflammation of the nerve as it passes through the abductor hallucis. MRI is the most useful modality for evaluating plantar pain. Coronal and sagittal T2-weighted images are most effective.

Posterior Pain

Posterior heel pain may be related to Achilles tendon injury or inflammation or bursitis. The first two were discussed previously. Retrocalcaneal burisitis is an inflammation of the bursa located between the Achilles and posterosuperior calcaneus. Patients with increased calcaneal inclination or cavus foot are more likely to be affected.

Lateral Pain

Lateral heel pain occurs infrequently. Peroneal tendon injury, described above, and sural nerve entrapment should be considered in this setting. Nerve entrapment may be caused by tendon sheath ganglia or avulsion fractures that cause entrapment of the nerve, which runs posterior to the peroneal tendons. MRI in the axial and sagittal planes is most useful for imaging this region.

Medial Pain

Medial tendon injuries were described previously. Tarsal tunnel syndrome is caused by irritation of the tibial nerve as it passes beneath the flexor retinaculum. Chronic trauma due to recurrent sprains and fractures or fracture dislocations may lead to tarsal tunnel syndrome.

Patients typically present with burning pain medially or heelparesthesia. Symptoms increase with weight bearing. MRI is most useful for evaluation of this and other medial hindfoot syndromes. Axial and sagittal T2-weighted images are most useful in this regard.

Forefoot Pain

Forefoot pain is a common problem in athletes. Those conditions responsible for these symptoms, excluding fractures, are reviewed below.

- Metatarsalgia: Metatarsal pain may be due to a long second metatarsal and a hypermobile first metatarsal. This localized form of forefoot pain usually correlates with a metatarsal pad insert. More generalized metatarsal pain is evident in athletes with a tight Achilles tendon or anterior ankle impingement. Surgical correction may be required in the latter.
- Sesamoiditis: Sesamoid pain syndromes are common in runners. The mdeial and lateral hallucis brevis. Their function is to elevate the first metatarsal head to disperse impact forces, to protect the flexor hallucis tendon, and to increase the

mechanical advantage of the flexor hallucis brevis tendon. The sesamoids may become inflamed or fractured or may undergo osteonecrosis. Patients with simple sesamioiditis usually respond to rest and longitudinal arch support. For those who do not respond, more significant injury must be excluded.

- Osteochondritis: Forefoot pain in athletes may also be due to osteonecrosis of the metatarsal head. The second metatarsal head is most commonly involved. Women are affected more frequently than men.
- Metatarsophalangeal subluxation and synovitis: Synovitis and/or subluxation of the metatarsophalangeal joints results in local tenderness, swelling, and pain with passive flexion. Synovitis is common in football players, especially those playing on artificial surfaces. The second metatarsophalangeal joint is most commonly affected; it is followed in frequency by the first and third joints. If the condition persists, hammertoe or medial or lateral translocation may develop. Subluxation more often occurs in middle-aged male joggers; the second metatarsal is most commonly involved. Other forefoot pain syndromes, neuromas, and stress fractures must be excluded.
- Hallux rigidus: Athletes frequently develop hallux rigidus, usually as a result of chronic trauma. Symptoms usually occur with starting from a squatting stance, such as in football or track. Hard-soled shoes may be helpful. In certain cases surgical correction may be indicated.
- Neuromas: Neuromas are due to chronic trauma to the interdigital nerve. Symptoms are commonly noted between the third and fourth metatarsal heads. Paresthesia and numbness is the sensory

distribution of the nerve are common. On examination, pain is elicited by placing pressure on the plantar aspect of the foot while compressing the metatarsal heads. Generally, properly fitting footwear or direct injection with anaesthetic and steroid will be successful. Surgery may be required in certain cases, however. In this setting, imaging is useful before consideration and planning of surgery.

Imaging of forefoot problems should begin with radiographs in the oblique and standing AP and lateral projections. Normal angles, joint congruency, and phalangeal deformities provide valuable clues to injury or foot deformities such as cavus foot that predispose to certain pain syndromes. The position and appearance of the sesamoids should be carefully assessed. Sesamoid are useful in patients with suspected abnormalities.

When routine radiographs are normal, radionuclide scans are useful to define early injuries such as stress fractures, sesamoiditis, or early osteonecrosis. Findings on bone scan can allow more specific imaging with CT or tomoraphy to define the lesion more effectively. Recently, MRI has become a frequent second choice after routine films. MRI can clearly define soft tissue lesions such as neuromas as well as osseous abnormalities.

Ankle Fractures

Management of foot and ankle fractures is a common problem for orthopaedic surgeons, emergency department physicians, family practice physicians, and radiologists. Imaging plays an important role in assessing the degree of bone and soft tissue injury and in following the healing process.

The detection of most fractures is not difficult. Detection of subtle fractures and evaluation of the extent ot soft tissue injury, however, may be more difficult. Thus it is essential for those interpreting images to be aware of the manner in which various fractures and soft tissue injuries present so that the images can be evaluated correctly and thoroughly. Soft tissue changes may be the only clue to a subtle fracture of ligament rupture. Soft tissue swelling, obliteration of the fat planes or the pre-Achilles fat triangle, and the presence of an effusion can be useful in identifying the location of subtle fractures.

It is also important to understand the clinical significance of certain fracture patterns. Fractures may be complete or incomplete. The latter are more common in children. Avulsion fractures occur at the insertion of ligaments or tendons.

Pediatric Ankle Fractures

Ankle fractures may be simple or complex with associated ligament rupture. The latter are more common in adults. Generally, fractures in patients older than 15 to 16 years of age are classified and treated on the basis of adult criteria.

The appearance of ankle fractures in children depends upon the age, relationship of the ligaments to the epiphytes, and mechanisms of injury. Distal diaphyseal and metaphyseal fractures are frequently incomplete. In most cases there is a posterior cortical break with buckling of the anterior cortex above the growth plate. Fractures of the distal tibia and fibula frequently involve the growth plates. The distal tibia epiphysis is the second most common site for growth plate fracture. In Rogers' series, 25% of 118 physeal injuries involved the distal tibia or fibula. Physeal fractures can result in growth or articular deformity if proper diagnosis and treatment are not implemented.

There are two types of epiphyses. Pressure epiphyses are located in the ends of long bones and are subject to weight-bearing forces and forces acting on the joint. Traction epiphyses occur at sites of muscle or tendon insertions. The latter are not directly associated with weight bearing. The pressure epiphyses of the distal tibia and fibula contribute 45% and 40%, respectively, of the growth of the tibia and fibula. The proximal epiphyses of the tibia contribute 55%, and those of the proximal fibula contribute 60%. The distal tibial and fibular epiphyses appear at age 2. The tibial epiphysis fuses by age 15 in girls and 17 in boys. The fibular epiphysis remains open longer and fuses at age 20.

Histologically the growth plate is divided into four zones. Progressing distally from the metaphysis, these zones include the zone of provisional calcification, the hypertrophic cartilage zone, the proliferating zone, and the resting zone. The cartilage cells are surrounded by longitudinally oriented collagen fibres and a chondrotin sulfate matrix. This substance is less abundant in the hypertrophic zone, which at least partially explains why this zone is the most susceptible to fracture. The blood supply to the epiphysis and metaphysis of the long bones is separate, with the exception of the proximal readial and femoral epiphyses. Therefore, when fracture of the growth plate occurs the blood supply is generally not disrupted. This spares the proliferating zone, and normal growth can occur after healing.

The same forces the cause fracture and/or ligament disruption in adults also cause fractures in children. In children the growth plates are two to five times weaker than the ligaments, so that fractures of the physes occur more commonly than ligament injuries. The fracture patterns that evolve are thus related to age, the ligamentous attachments, and the type of force applied.

Growth plate fractures are more common during the first year and the rapid growth phases in the early teens.

The most commonly used classification system for physical injuries was described by Salter and Harris. This classification is useful because of its prognostic significance and easy-to-use radiographic patterns. Type I fractures are due to separation of the epiphysis with the fracture line confined to the growth plate. The fracture usually extends through the hypertrophic zone and does not involve the epiphysis or metaphysis. In Rogers' of injury may be subtle radiographically. Comparison radiographs of the uninjured ankle may be helpful. Type I injuries are uncommon in athletes and tend to occur more commonly in children younger than 5 years of age. The prognosis is generally excellent.

Type II fractures are the most common. This fracture extends through the growth plate for a variable distance before exiting through the metaphysis. Type II fractures occur more commonly in patients older than 10 years of age. Eversion or inversion injuries with forced abduction or adduction of the foot have been implicated in this ankle fracture.

Type III fractures are intraarticular, extending through the epiphysis and entering the growth plate, where they exit through the hypertrophic zone. The metaphysis is spared. This injury is usually due to an intraarticular shearing force.

Type IV fractures extend from the articular surface of the epiphysis through the growth plate and exit through the metaphysis. Complete reduction of this fracture is essential to prevent growth disturbances. This fracture makes up 10% of Salter-Harris fractures.

Type V fractures are the result of compression injuries that cause impaction of the growth plate. The ankle and knee are commonly involved. The prognosis is guarded with type V fractures. These tractures are uncommon.

Other classifications have also been applied to growth plate fractures. Crensnaw proposed a classification similar to that of Salter and Harris that is frequently used because of its simplicity. Injuries are categorized according to forces applied: external rotation, abduction, adduction, plantar flexion, and direct trauma. With this approach the pattern of injury can be used in fracture reduction. Fractures are reduced by gently reversing the direction of the mechanism of injury noted radiographically.

External rotation injuries occur when the foot is subjected to external rotation forces. This tress leads to fracture of the posterolateral tibial physis and often a fracture of the fibula above the growth plate. Abduction injuries result in Salter-Harris I or II fractures of the anterolateral tibia. The direction of stress and talar shift usually displaces the fragment laterally. Talar forces may lead to associated fibular fractures. Adduction forces are similar to inversion injuries, placing tension on the lateral ligament complex. This results in avulsion or distal fibular physical fractures. The force, if continued, will cause impaction of the talus against the medial malleolus, leading to a Salter-Harris III or IV fracture of the medial malleolus. Plantar flexion injuries lead to posterior epiphyseal injuries. By definition there is no external rotation force, and therefore no associated fibular fracture is evident. The Crenshaw fracture patterns are most common during the 12th year, and there is a significantly higher incidence in boys.

More recently, the Lauge-Hansen system has been combined with the Salter-Harris system. The former is an accurate method commonly applied to adult ankle injuries and is discussed later. Dias and Tachdjian studied 71 patients with their combined classification system, and only 4 patients did not properly fit the categories. This classification, like the Lauge-Hansen system, is based on the position of the foot during the injury and the direction of the abnormal force.

Several ankle fractures do not fit into this classification. A Salter-Harris III of the distal tibia is usually due to external rotation forces. This fracture is generally seen in the lateral portion of the tibia. Triplane is generally seen in the lateral portion of the tibia. Triplanc fractures do not fit the original Dias-Tachdjian classification. The injury is believed to be due to external rotation with or without associated plantar flexion. The fracture consists of three fragments instead of the two fragments seen with most growth plate fractures. The first fragment involves the anterolateral portion of the tibial epiphysis and looks like a Salter-Harris III injury. The second fragment is the remainder of the tibial epiphysis with the metaphyseal attachment. The third fragment is the tibial metaphysis. The fracture has a characteristic radiographic appearance. On the AP view it has the appearance. On the AP view it has the appearance of a Salter-Harris III fracture, and on the lateral view it resembles a Salter-Harris II fracture of the distal tibia. The incidence of triplane fractures is not high. Cooperman et al noted an incidence of 6% in a series of 237 patients with epiphyseal fractures of the ankle. In reality the fracture behaves like a Salter-Harris IV, and since its original description many investigators hold that it is often only a two-part fracture. The medial malleolus and anteromedial portion of the epiphysis remain attached to the tibial metaphysis and form one fragment. The second fragment is the lateral portion of the epiphysis with the lateral metaphysical attachment.

Other variations of he triplance fracture have also been described.

The so-called juvenile Tillaux fracture is a Salter-Harris III fracture of the distal lateral tibia. The fragment is displaced by the distal tibiofibular ligaments when the foot is externally rotated.

Most epiphysical injuries can be clearly defined on the routine ankle trauma series: AP, lateral, and morise views. In most cases the entire tibia and fibula should be included on the films so that a high fibular fracture is not overlooked. Fractures of the fibular physis, the most common ankle fracture, may be very subtle. Usually Salter-Harris I or, more commonly, II fractures are best seen on the mortise view. When the foot is internally rotated 15° to 20°, the fibula is viewed clear of the tibia. This fracture, however, should be suspected in any child with swelling and point tenderness over the growth plate. When no other fractures are evident the patient can be splinted, and a repeat study in 10 to 14 days will often demonstrate the fracture line more clearly. Slight perosteal callus may also be evident at this time. When a Salter-Harris III or IV fracture is present medially, one should assume that the growth plate or the lateral ligaments are damaged or that an avulsion fracture may be present. Salter-Harris I and II fractures of the distal tibia may also present with subtle radiographic findings. Comparison views on an approach similar to the one described above can be used to evaluate these fractures.

More complex physical injuries, especially triplane fractures or comminuted epiphyseal fractures, can be better evaluated with CT or MRI. These techniques clearly demonstrate the epiphyseal fragmentation and distal tibiofibular relationships. As is the case for adults, it is important to define the degree of articular involvement, note any articular irregularity, and clearly define the degree of separation of the fracture fragments. Displacement of more than 2 mm has significant treatment implications.

Adult Ankle Fractures

Complete evaluation of ankle fractures in adults includes assessment of the fracture fragments and accurate description of associated ligament injuries. Evaluation of bone and soft tissue involvement is important in determining the mechanism of injury, which in turn has significant treatment implications.

When evaluating ankle fractures it is common to consider the bones and ligaments a ring-like structure in the coronal plane. The ring is made up of the medial malleolus, tibial plafond, distal tibiofibular ligaments and syndemosis, lateral malleolus, lateral ligaments, talus, and medial ligaments. Breaks in the ring commonly occur at five sites either alone or in combination. Shift of the talus indicates disruption of the ring at more than one site. The five common sites of injury include the lateral malleolus, lateral ligaments, deltoid ligaments, medial malleolus, and syndesmosis. Fractures of the tibial plafond occur after axial loading with various degrees of plantar flexion.

Clinical Features

After ankle injury, patients generally present with various degrees of pain, swelling, and ecchymosis depending to some degree on the significance of the injury. The incidence of swelling and presence of ecchymosis is somewhat higher when fractures are present, but this is not a reliable clinical finding. With incomplete injuries and stable fractures weight bearing is usually still possible. Weight bearing is more difficult or impossible with unstable fractures.

Most ankle fractures occur as a result of inversion or eversion forces. The mechanism of injury is rarely pure, however. Most often abduction, adduction, lateral rotation, of axial loading occur in addition to eversion or inversion.

The value of classifications for ankle fractures is that they have a significant impact on treatment, prognosis, and establishing the mechanism of injury. Classifications must also be workable and easy to remember. With this in mind, various classifications have been developed for ankle fractures. The more commonly employed classifications are those proposed by Lauge-Hansen and Weber. The former is accurate in predicting the mechanism of injury and extent of ligament involvement. Therefore, it is recommended to radiologists so that the description of the injury can be most accurate. The Weber classification is not as complex but is frequently used because of its value in planning apprcpriate therapy.

The Lauge-Hansen classification was devised with the use of cadaver specimens. It is based on the position of the foot at the time of injury and the direction of the injuring force. With this system, four basic categorise of injury are described. The classification considers different levels of injury in each category on the basis of the degree of the force and the length of time for which it is applied.

Supination-adduction injuries cause traction on the lateral ligaments, resulting in either a ligament tear of an avulsion fracture of the lateral malleolus. The fracture is generally transverse and below the joint level. If the force is sufficient, the talus can impact against the medial malleolus. If an oblique fracture of the medial malleolus is evident but not fracture is seen in the lateral malleolus, one can assume that the lateral ligaments are disrupted.

PREVENTIVE MEASURES

1. Wear the correct shoes for your particular activity.

2. Wear hiking shoes or boots in rough terrain.

3. Don't continue to wear any sports shoe if it is worn unevenly

4. The toe box in "steel-toe" shoes should be deep enough to accommodate your toes comfortably.

5. Always wear hard-top shoes when operating a lawn mower or other grass-cutting equipment.

6. Don't walk barefoot on paved streets or sidewalks.

7. Watch out for slippery floors at home and at work. Clean up obviously dangerous spills immediately.

8. If you get up during the night, turn on a light. Many fractured toes and other foot injuries occur while attempting to find one's way in the dark.

9

CARE AND PREVENTION OF HEAD INJURIES

Head injuries can occur in any sport and in a variety of ways. However, most head injuries are caused by the application of some type of sudden force to the head. This sudden force is usually the result of a direct blow. Trauma of this type may be caused by the athlete colliding with another athlete or object such as a goal post, wall, bleacher, or the floor or ground. It may also occur if the athlete is struck by some sort of athletic equipment, such as a baseball bat or hockey stick. In addition, the head may be injured by a blow from a projectile such as a baseball, golf ball, discus, or hockey puck. The face or cervical spine may also be injured as a result of 'such sudden" force.

The term "head injury" may be used to describe damage to the scalp, skull, brain. It is important to realize, however, that all three of these structures may not be damaged in anyone injury. For example, it is possible for a skull fracture to occur with little or no injury to either the scalp or the brain. As a matter of fact, most head injuries occurring in .athletics are not associated with a skill fracture.

The scalp protects the skull. Without this protection, the skull could be fractured or the brain injured by much less force. It is important to understand the anatomy of the scalp because injury or infection to the scalp can also involve the skull or brain.

Head Injury Overview

Head injury is a general term used to describe any trauma to the head, and most specifically to the brain itself.

Skull fracture: A skull fracture is a break in the bone surrounding the brain and other structures within the skull.

Linear skull fracture: A common injury, especially in children. A linear skull fracture is a simple break in the skull that follows a relatively straight line. It can occur after seemingly minor head injuries (falls, blows such as being struck by a rock, stick, or other object; or from motor vehicle accidents). A linear skull fracture is not a serious injury unless there is an additional injury to the brain itself.

Depressed skull fractures: These are common after forceful impact by blunt objects-most commonly, hammers, rocks, or other heavy but fairly small objects. These injuries cause "dents" in the skull bone. If the depth of a depressed fracture is at least equal to the thickness of the surrounding skull bone (about 1/4-1/2 inch), surgery is often required to elevate the bony pieces and to inspect the brain for evidence of injury. Minimally depressed fractures are less than the thickness of the bone. Other fractures are not depressed at all. They usually do not require surgical treatment unless other injuries are noted.

Basilar skull fracture: A fracture of the bones that form the base (floor) of the skull and results from severe blunt head trauma of significant force. A basilar skull fracture commonly connects to the sinus cavities. This connection may allow fluid or air entry into the inside of the skull and may cause infection. Surgery is usually not necessary unless other injuries are also involved.

Intracranial (inside the skull) hemorrhage (bleeding)

Subdural hematoma: Bleeding between the brain tissue and the dura mater (a tough fibrous layer of tissue between the brain and skull) is called a subdural hematoma. The stretching and tearing of "bridging veins" between the brain and dura mater causes this type of bleeding. A subdural hematoma may be acute, developing suddenly after the injury, or chronic, slowly accumulating after injury. Chronic subdural hematoma is more common in the elderly whose bridging veins are often brittle and stretched and can more easily begin to slowly bleed after minor injuries. Subdural hematomas are potentially serious and may require surgery.

Epidural hematoma: The skull is made up of a variety of bones; the dura, the thick membrane that wraps around the brain, attaches at the suture lines where the bones come together. If bleeding occurs in the enclosed space between the dura and the bone, and a hematoma (blood clot) forms, there is nowhere for it to accumulate and pressure within the epidural space can build quickly. The increasing pressure pushes the hematoma against the brain tissue and may cause significant damage.

Tiny epidural hematomas potentially may be observed without surgery, but often surgery is indicated to removed the hematoma and relieve the pressure on the brain. The earlier the operation, the better, because the death rate increases if the patient is in a coma at the time of operation.

An epidural hematoma may often occur with trauma to the temporal bone located on the side of the head above the ear. Aside from the fact that the temporal bone is thinner than the other skull bones (frontal, parietal, occipital), it is also the location of the middle meningeal artery that runs just beneath the bone. Fracture of the temporal bone is associated with tearing of this artery and may lead to an epidural hematoma.

Subarachnoid hemorrhage: Subarachnoid hemorrhage can be caused by trauma and often does not require surgery. Blood accumulates in the space beneath the arachnoid layer that surrounds the brain. While this can irritate the brain and cause symptoms of headache, vomiting, and stiff neck, treatment may be watchful waiting without surgery unless symptoms worsen.

Intraparenchymal hemorrhage/cerebral contusion: These terms describe bleeding into the brain tissue itself. A contusion is like a bruise to the brain tissue and usually requires no special intervention, much like a concussion. Most doctors admit people with cerebral (brain) contusion to the hospital for observation since there may be rare complications such as brain swelling. An intraparenchymal hemorrhage is a pool of blood within the brain tissue. Minor bleeding may stop without any treatment and cause no serious problems. More serious or large bleeds usually require surgery.

Closed head injuries: This broad term describes any injury to the brain or structures within the skull that is not caused by a penetrating injury (such as a gunshot wound or stab wound). They range from very minor to potentially fatal injuries.

HEAD INJURY CAUSES

All types of head injuries can be caused by trauma. In adults in the United States such injuries commonly result from motor vehicle accidents, assaults, and falls. In children falls are the most common cause followed by recreational activities such as biking, skating, or skateboarding. A small but significant number of head injuries in children are from violence and abuse.

Penetrating trauma: Missiles such as bullets or sharp instruments (such as knives, screwdrivers, or ice picks) may penetrate the skull. The result is called a penetrating head injury. Penetrating injuries often require surgery to remove debris from the brain tissue. The initial injury itself may cause immediate death, especially if from a high-energy missile such as a bullet.

Blunt head trauma: These injuries may be from a direct blow (a club or large missile) or from a rapid deceleration force (a fall or striking the windshield in a car accident).

Head injuries are potentially the most serious athletic injuries. Although fatalities in sports are relatively rare, injuries to the head account for more fatalities than injuries to any other area of the body. Permanently disabling brain damage resulting from athletic activity is also rare. However, injuries to the brain do occur, and no head injury should be treated lightly. Anyone who has the responsibility of caring for athletic injuries should plan and prepare for devastating injury. Head injuries can produce a wide array of complex symptoms, and correct assessment procedures by the athletic trainer are extremely important.

PRIMARY SURVEY :

(a) Airway

(b) Breathing

(c) Circulation

The importance of maintaining airway, breathing and circulation are important. These important steps of basic life support can never be neglected with any athletic injury. Always check and continue to monitor an athlete's airway, breathing and circulation throughout the assessment process to recognize and correct any life-threatening problems. Whenever an injured athlete is responsive, the primary survey can be completed quickly and with little difficulty.

SECONDARY SURVEY : NEUROLOGIC BASELINE

Neurologic baseline gives the athletic trainer and the physician a clue for further investigation. If the athlete improves from this baseline, there is a good chance that there is no additional intracranial involvement. Remember that intracranial involvement may take a period of time to develop. An athlete may appear to be doing fine immediately after an injury and then develop signs and symptoms hours later. An important aspect of the assessment of a head-injured athlete is the manner in which physical signs and symptoms progress. This is why it is important to do repeated evaluations over a period of time with an athlete who suffers an injury to the head. Physical changes are only appreciated if the athlete's initial status is evaluated and documented. When an athlete's condition deteriorates from the original neurologic baseline, it suggests additional intracranial involvement; he or she must be referred for medical assistance. This baseline information is extremely important to the physician who must diagnose the severity of injury after referral. It is, unfortunately, often neglected in the rush to get an injured athlete to medical assistance. Neurologic information should always be written down and reported to the physician. In reporting your evaluations, it is better to describe your findings in functional language. For example, to use a term such as "lethargic" is subject to misinterpretations. It is better to report the athlete's actions or behavior; for example "the athlete responded accurately to verbal commands but would then fall asleep."

Always handle the athlete with a head injury as

though he or she has a cervical spine injury until proved otherwise. This includes protecting the injured athlete from any unnecessary movement during the assessment process. If movement of the athlete is necessary for any reason, absolute control of the head is essential.

Secondary survey gives enough information on an athlete who has suffered an injury to the head. Throughout the evaluation process look for signs and symptoms that may indicate the athlete has an expanding intracranial lesion or cervical spine involvement. Whenever any of these signs are recognized. It is not necessary to continue the assessment. It is time to seek medical assistance for the athlete. This point must be remembered and cannot be overemphasized.

History

A brief history for those injuries involving the head will be helpful Gain as much information surrounding the circumstances of the injury as possible. Attempt to determine the mechanism of injury and direction of force. Following question may be asked.

(1) Was there a loss of consciousness.

(2) Did the athlete have, a seizure?

(3) Does the athlete have any medical problems that may be associated with the injury?

Details of the injury, as well as specific time intervals between any changing clinical signs, should be recorded because this information is invaluable for diagnosis. Obtain as much information as possible from the injured athlete. Many symptoms may not be volunteered by the injured athlete but must be actively sought through questioning. If the athlete cannot remember or is stuporous or uncooperative, attempt to obtain information from anyone who witnessed the injury.

Note the level of consciousness of the injured athlete and then ascertain any subsequent changes. In most instances the athlete's level of consciousness will improve in a short period of time. If the athlete regains consciousness quickly, the prognosis for a rapid and uneventful recovery is good. If the athlete regains consciousness slowly, the prognosis is more guarded. The athlete who shows minimal or very slow improvement should be referred to a physician or medical facility-A decrease in the level of consciousness is the most sensitive indicator of additional intracranial involvement; anytime the level of consciousness deteriorates, immediate medical attention is indicated.

SYMPTOMS

1. HEADACHE

Headache is another frequent symptom of a head injury. A headache that becomes- progressively more severe is an alarming symptom that may indicate additional intracranial involvement. The persistence of a headache indicates that whatever damage occurred to the brain has not subsided, and the athlete should not return to activity The cessation of the headache is probably the most reliable indicator that adequate recovery has occurred and the athlete can return to activity, providing also that there are no other positive neurologic signs

(1) As you periodically check on the health status of an athlete who has suffered an injury to the head.

(2) Remember to question the athlete about his or her headache. In addition to the mechanism of injury, level of consciousness, and headache, you should attempt to gain further information during the history

portion of the assessment process.

Question the athlete about his or her feelings

(1) Concerning the head and neck.

(2) Is there any pain in the neck?

(3) Does the athlete feel any numbness, weakness, or tingling?

(4) Does the athlete complain of any ringing in the ears (tinnitus), dizziness, nausea, or blurred or double vision?

All this information is important in establishing a neurologic baseline and should be obtained by talking with the injured athlete. In addition, question the athlete about any other painful or tender areas of the body that my require further evaluation.

An athlete suffering from a head injury requires close observation throughout the assessment process. Watch the athlete carefully as you carry out the history-taking procedures. Notice if the athlete has any difficulty in finding or saying the right words or understanding commands (aphasia). Check for any obvious deformities or abnormal positions of any body athlete attempts any movements of the head, neck, or extremities the athlete demonstrate any weakness or paralysis? Watch for neurologic signs that may indicate the existence of expanding intracranial pressure, such as pilary signs, irregular respirations, seizures, or a decreasing level of consciousness.

SIGNS

1. Level of consciousness

Establishing and monitoring the level of consciousness is the most important neurologic sign to be gained during the assessment of a head injury.

Question the athlete in an attempt to evaluate the level of alertness, responsiveness, awareness, and orientation. Begin by checking the athletes awareness to person, place, and time. Can the athlete answer simple questions such as "What is your name? Where are you?' 'How old are you?" "Do you know who I am?" Then ask the athlete questions that require more thought, such as "What do you do on a certain play?" Questioning along this line may require the assistance of a coach or another player who is aware of the correct answers. Also evaluate the athlete's memory. Can the athlete remember the events leading up to the injury? What was the first recollection following the injury? The severity of the injury is many times proportional to the lack of memory; that is, the longer the period of amnesia, the greater the injury to the brain.

2. Pupils

Both pupils should be symmetric in size and react quickly and equally to light. When one pupil becomes larger and shows a decreased response to light, there is strong evidence for increased intracranial pressure: The athlete should be referred to a physician Also observe the eye movements. Normally the eyes gaze straight ahead, unless focused on something. The movement of the eyes should be coordinated; with a head injury, the gaze may be abnormal, or the eyes may turn in different directions. Any abnormal, uncoordinated, or involuntary movement of the eyes may indicate intracranial involvement. If the athlete is conscious, instruct him or her to follow your finger with the eyes and notice whether eye movement is paralyzed or decreased in any direction. For example, an athlete with a fracture of the orbit is usually not able to look upward as far on the fractured side. Involuntary rapid movement of the eyeballs in any direction (nystagmus) is another indication of intracranial involvement.

3. Respirations

A normal respiratory pattern suggests that there is no apparent brain damage, at least at that time. Abnormal breathing patterns may indicate severe brain dysfunction and the need for medical assistance. Look for any signs of trauma, which can give important clues as to the nature and severity of the injury. Examine the head, neck, and face for any deformities, lacerations, contusions, or hemorrhaging. Cuts and bruises are reliable signs that strong forces have been applied to the athletes head. Watch for any discharge coming from the ears or nose. Look for unusual or abnormal positions of any part of the body, which may indicate any additional injuries

4. Palpation

Much of the information necessary to establish a neurologic baseline will be gained during the history and observation portion of the assessment process. However, once the injured athlete is stable, additional information can be gained through gender palpation. It is important to evaluate the rate and nature of the pulse in an athlete who has suffered an injury to the head. The pulse should be felt periodically during the evaluation.

HEAD INJURY SYMPTOMS

Signs and symptoms of head injuries vary with the type and severity of the injury.

Minor blunt head injuries may involve only symptoms of being "dazed" or brief loss of consciousness. They may result in headaches or blurring of vision or nausea and vomiting. There may be longer lasting subtle symptoms including, irritability, difficulty concentrating, insomnia, and difficulty tolerating bright light and loud sounds. These post concussion symptoms may last for a prolonged period of time.

Severe blunt head trauma involves a loss of consciousness lasting from several minutes to many days or longer. Seizures may result. The person may suffer from severe and sometimes permanent neurological deficits or may die. Neurological deficits from head trauma resemble those seen in stroke and include paralysis, seizures, or difficulty with speaking, seeing, hearing, walking, or understanding.

Penetrating trauma may cause immediate, severe symptoms or only minor symptoms despite a potentially life-threatening injury. Death may follow from the initial injury. Any of the signs of serious blunt head trauma may result.

WHEN TO SEEK MEDICAL CARE

Emergency personnel should immediately attend to all potentially serious head injuries.

Call the doctor to ask about any of the following situations. Your doctor will recommend home care, set up an appointment to see you, or direct you to go to a hospital's Emergency Department.

- A person is pushed to the ground or struck a hard object with the head but did not lose consciousness
- Vomiting more than once
- Confusion
- Drowsiness
- Weakness or inability to walk

Severe headache

Go to the Emergency Department by ambulance in

the following situations. People with less severe injuries may be taken by car to the Emergency Department.

- Severe head trauma or a fall from more than the height of the person or a hard fall onto a hard surface or object.

- Loss of consciousness for more than 1 minute, vomiting more than once, confusion, drowsiness, weakness or inability to walk, or severe headache

- Prevent movement of the neck in severe head injury or if the injured person has any neck pain. If the person needs to vomit, carefully roll them onto their side without turning the head.

- Should an injured person be allowed to fall asleep? Many people mistakenly believe that it is important to keep a person awake after they have been struck on the head. Children often are more emotionally disturbed than they are physically injured after a minor fall. They will cry and be upset, but as the parent rushes them to the hospital, the child may begin to calm down. They have expended a lot of physical and emotional energy by crying and then will often want to fall asleep.

- You do not need to keep a child or other victim of head injury awake. In many cases it is even helpful to the emergency doctor to be able to awaken a child who is now calm and rested and able to behave normally. This gives the doctor a much better assessment of the severity of the head injury.

- If a person who was initially normal after a head injury cannot be awakened or is extremely difficult to awaken, he or she may have a more serious head injury and should be evaluated by a doctor.

HEAD INJURY TREATMENT

Self-Care at Home

Emergency medical personnel should immediately treat any serious or potentially serious head injury.

Minor head injuries may be cared for at home.

Bleeding under the scalp, but outside the skull, creates "goose eggs" or large bruises at the site of a head injury. They are common and will go away on their own with time. Using ice immediately after the trauma may help decrease their size.

Do not apply ice directly to the skin. Ice should be applied for 20-30 minutes at a time and can be repeated about every 2-4 hours as needed.

Use a light washcloth as a barrier and wrap the ice in it. You can also use a bag of frozen vegetables wrapped in cloth. This conforms nicely to the shape of the head.

Make your own ice pack by adding 1/3 cup of 70% isopropyl alcohol (the green-colored kind is best to help identify it later) to 2/3 cup of water in a zip-lock-style bag (double bag it to prevent leaking). The mixture turns into "slush." Freeze this homemade ice pack for use when needed. Caution: If you have small children in your home, watch them carefully when using the ice pack. Drinking the mixture can be poisonous.

Commercially available ice packs use chemicals to create cold. They are designed to be kept in a first-aid kit and need not be kept frozen. These can be applied directly to the skin, although a barrier can also be used if bleeding is present. They must be disposed of after a single use but can be handy in case of emergencies.

When a minor head injury results from a fall onto carpet or other soft surface and the height of the fall is less than the height of the person who fell and there is no loss of consciousness (in other words, the person was not "knocked out"), a doctor's visit is not usually needed. Apply ice to lessen swelling.

MEDICAL TREATMENT

Treatment varies widely depending on the type and severity of injuries.

• Minor head injuries are often treated at home as long as someone is available to watch the person.

• Bed rest, fluids, and a mild pain reliever, for example, acetaminophen (Tylenol) may be prescribed. Ice may be applied to the scalp for pain relief and to decrease swelling.

• Cuts will be numbed with a medication usually given by injection. They will then be cleansed. The doctor will then look for foreign matter and hidden injuries. The wound usually is closed with skin staples, stitches (sutures), or skin glue. Tetanus immunization will be updated if needed.

• People with serious closed head injuries are almost always admitted to the hospital for observation and repeated studies to assure that the condition does not worsen.

• Occasionally a head injury may cause elevated pressure within the skull. An intracranial pressure (ICP) monitor probe may be surgically inserted into the brain through the skull to measure the pressure. If the pressure rises too high, it may be necessary to do surgery to decompress the brain. Death is possible. Intravenous medications may be used to control intracranial pressure as a temporizing measure until the crisis resolves or surgery is performed.

• Medication to prevent seizures may be given to prevent or treat seizures that occur from the head injury. Seizures after head injury often do not require treatment because they may not reoccur.

• Antibiotics are usually not required in closed head injuries. Some doctors use antibiotics in all cases of basilar skull fracture. Other doctors do not feel this is useful.

• When there is a closed head injury with bleeding inside the skull, the doctor must consider a number of factors to determine the correct treatment. Some of these include the location of the bleeding, severity of the symptoms, the presence of any other injuries, and progression of symptoms. Surgery may be needed. Other options include pressure monitors, medication to prevent seizures, and antibiotics to prevent infection. People with this type of injury may need a breathing tube inserted (intubation) to help prevent further brain injury. Angiography may be performed.

• Penetrating head injuries often require some sort of surgery, usually to remove foreign material or to stop bleeding. Other options include pressure monitors, medication to prevent seizures, and antibiotics to prevent infection. People with this type of injury may need a breathing tube inserted. Angiography may be performed.

NEXT STEPS

Prevention

• Sensible prevention includes wearing helmets when bike riding, inline skating, driving motorcycles, and other similar activities.

• Safety belts, car seats, and airbags when used

properly can prevent head injuries in motor vehicle accidents.

• Drinking while driving is one of the most common causes of motor vehicle crashes. Many serious head injuries would be prevented by avoiding this dangerous behavior.

• Fall-proofing includes checking your home for areas where someone may fall: stairs, bathtubs, throw rugs, and furniture.

10

CARE AND PREVENTION OF HAND AND WRIST INJURIES

The hand, which includes the fingers and thumb, is a functionally intricate and complex anatomic structure located at the distal end of our upper extremity. The wrist is that area of articulation between the forearm and hand. Precise functioning of the hand and wrist is essential to almost every type of athletic activity. The primary function of the proximal portion of the upper extremity is to position the hand where it can best perform its designated tasks. Functional anatomists sometimes refer to the hand and wrist as the "reason for the upper extremity." Both structures are frequently used during athletic activity and often function as a single unit. Together they permit an incredible array of intricate movements and also serve to absorb or transmit forces caused by falls or traumatic contact. Because the hand and wrist normally do not bear weight and because injuries to this area are not usually totally disabling, there is a tendency by some athletes to underestimate the severity and importance of these injuries. Many injuries to the hand and wrist are relatively minor and do not require extensive care. However, if neglected or unrecognized, they can develop into long-term impairment and possibly permanent disability and disfigurement. Hand and wrist injuries may require expert treatment to avoid these complications. It is imperative therefore that athletic trainers be able to accurately assess athletic injuries to this important area of the body, initiate proper treatment, and recognize when referral is necessary. The comprehensive evaluation of injuries to the hand and wrist begins with a well-founded knowledge of grass and functional anatomy of the area as well as an understanding of the common athletic injuries and how they may occur.

Finger, hand, or wrist injuries most commonly occur during:

- Sports or recreational activities.
- Work-related tasks.
- Work or projects around the home, especially if using machinery such as lawn mowers, snow blowers, or hand tools.
- Accidental falls.
- Fistfights.

The risk of finger, hand, or wrist injury is higher in contact sports, such as wrestling, football, or soccer, and in high-speed sports, such as biking, in-line skating, skiing, snowboarding, and skateboarding. Sports that require weight-bearing on the hands and arms, such as gymnastics, can increase the risk for injury. Sports that use hand equipment such as ski poles, hockey or lacrosse sticks, or racquets also increase the risk of injury.

In children, most finger, hand, or wrist injuries occur during sports or play or from accidental falls. Any injury occurring at the end of a long bone near a joint may injure the growth plate (physis) and needs to be evaluated.

Older adults are at higher risk for injuries and fractures, because they lose muscle mass and bone strength (osteopenia) as they age. They also have more problems with vision and balance, which increases their risk of accidental injury.

Most minor injuries will heal on their own, and home treatment is usually all that is needed to relieve symptoms and promote healing.

SUDDEN (ACUTE) INJURY

An acute injury may occur from a direct blow, a penetrating injury, or a fall, or from twisting, jerking, jamming, or bending a limb abnormally. Pain may be sudden and severe. Bruising and swelling may develop soon after the injury. Acute injuries include:

- **Bruises.** After a wrist or hand injury, bruising may extend to the fingers from the effects of gravity. See a picture of a bruise (contusion).
- **Injuries to ligaments.** See a picture of a torn thumb ligament as in skier's thumb.
- Injuries to tendons, such as mallet finger.
- Injuries to joints (sprains).
- Pulled muscles (strains).
- Broken bones (fractures), such as a wrist fracture.
- Dislocations.
- Crushing injury, which can lead to compartment syndrome.

OVERUSE INJURIES

Overuse injuries occur when too much stress is placed on a joint or other tissue, often by "overdoing" an activity or repeating the same activity. Overuse injuries include the following:

- **Carpal tunnel syndrome** is caused by pressure on a nerve (median nerve) in the wrist. The symptoms include tingling, numbness, weakness, or pain of the fingers and hand. See a picture of carpal tunnel syndrome.

- **Tendon pain** is actually a symptom of tendinosis, a series of very small tears (microtears) in the tissue in or around the tendon. In addition to pain and tenderness, common symptoms of tendon injury include decreased strength and movement in the affected area.

- **De Quervain's disease** can occur in the hand and wrist when tendons and the tendon covering (sheath) on the thumb side of the wrist swell and become inflamed. See a picture of de Quervain's disease.

Treatment

Treatment for a finger, hand, or wrist injury may include first aid measures; medicine; "buddy-taping" for support; application of a brace, splint, or cast; physical therapy; and in some cases, surgery. Treatment depends on:

- The location, type, and severity of the injury.
- How long ago the injury occurred.
- Your age, health condition, and activities (such as work, sports, or hobbies).

Review the Emergencies and Check Your Symptoms sections to determine if and when you need to see a doctor.

Emergencies

Do you have any of the following symptoms that require emergency treatment? Call 911 or other emergency services immediately.

- Signs of shock occur:

- In children.
- In adults and older children.
- Severe bleeding does not slow during the first 15 minutes of steady, direct pressure.
- Any part of your hand is partially or completely amputated. Begin first aid measures.
- Pieces of bone are visible in a wound, or a bone is sticking through the skin. Note: Do not try to push the bone back into the skin. Cover the area with a clean bandage.
- Injection of a substance under high pressure into the hand, such as paint from a high-pressure paint sprayer or a nail from a powered nail gun
- Severe pain with pale, white, blue, or cold fingers or hand

Check Your Symptoms

If you answer yes to any of the following questions, click on the "Yes" in front of the question for information about how soon to see a health professional.

Review health risks that may increase the seriousness of your symptoms.

If you have any of the following symptoms, evaluate those symptoms first.

- **Bleeding:** Go to the topic Cuts or Scrapes.
- Puncture wound or injection of a foreign body under high pressure: Go to the topic Puncture Wounds.
- A finger, hand, or wrist problem not related to an injury: Go to the topic Finger, Hand, and Wrist Problems, Noninjury.
- Injury from cold exposure: Go to the topic Cold

Temperature Exposure.

- A burn to a finger, hand, or wrist: Go to the topic Burns.

- A bite to a finger, hand, or wrist: Go to the topic Animal and Human Bites.

- A fingernail problem or blood under a nail: Go to the topic Nail Problems and Injuries.

HOME TREATMENT

First aid for a suspected broken bone

- If a bone is sticking out of the skin, do not try to push it back into the skin. Cover the area with a clean bandage.

- **Control bleeding.**

- Remove all bracelets or rings. It may be difficult to remove the jewelry once swelling occurs, which in turn can cause other serious problems, such as nerve compression or restricted blood flow. See a picture of removing a ring that is stuck.

- Free a trapped finger or hand from an object, such as a pipe, toy, or jar.

- Splint the injured area without trying to straighten the injured limb. Loosen the wrap around the splint if signs develop that indicate the wrap is too tight, such as numbness, tingling, increased pain, swelling, or cool skin below the wrap. A problem called compartment syndrome can develop.

- Home treatment for a sore or sprained finger

- Use rest, ice, compression, and elevation (RICE) for pain and swelling.

- If you do not have diabetes or peripheral arterial

disease, your sore or sprained finger can be " buddy-taped" to your uninjured finger next to it. Protect the skin by putting some soft padding, such as felt or foam, between your fingers before you tape them together. Your injured finger may need to be buddy-taped for 2 to 4 weeks to heal. If your injured finger hurts more after you have buddy taped it, remove the tape and use the Check Your Symptoms section to check your symptoms again. Caution: Never splint a finger in a completely straight position, such as on a Popsicle stick. For proper healing, the finger should be slightly bent and in a relaxed position.

- Stop, change, or take a break from activities that cause your symptoms.

- Home treatment for a minor hand or wrist injury

- Home treatment may help relieve pain, swelling, and stiffness.

- Remove all rings, bracelets, or any other jewelry that goes around a finger or wrist. It will be more difficult to remove the jewelry later if swelling increases.

- Use rest, ice, compression, and elevation (RICE) for pain and swelling.

- Do not use your injured hand or wrist for the first 24 hours after an injury, if possible. An elastic bandage can help decrease swelling. The wrap will also remind you to rest the injured hand or wrist. A wrist splint can help support an injured wrist. Talk to your doctor if you think you need to use a splint or bandage for more than 48 to 72 hours.

- Gently massage or rub the area to relieve pain and encourage blood flow. Do not massage the injured area if it causes pain.

- For the first 48 hours after an injury, avoid things

that might increase swelling, such as hot showers, hot tubs, hot packs, or alcoholic beverages.

- After 48 to 72 hours, if swelling is gone, apply heat and begin gentle exercise with the aid of moist heat to help restore and maintain flexibility. Some experts recommend alternating between heat and cold treatments.
- Treat blisters.

Safety tips

- Be sure to follow these safety tips when you use a nonprescription medicine:
- Carefully read and follow all directions on the medicine bottle and box.
- Do not take more than the recommended dose.
- Do not take a medicine if you have had an allergic reaction to it in the past.
- If you have been told to avoid a medicine, call your doctor before you take it.
- If you are or could be pregnant, do not take any medicine other than acetaminophen unless your doctor has told you to.
- Do not give aspirin to anyone younger than age 20 unless your doctor tells you to.
- Symptoms to Watch For During Home Treatment
- Use the Check Your Symptoms section to evaluate your symptoms if any of the following occur during home treatment.
- Pain or swelling develops.
- Signs of infection develop.
- Numbness; tingling; or cool, pale skin develops.

- Symptoms do not improve with home treatment.
- Symptoms become more severe or frequent.

Prevention

The following tips may prevent finger, hand, and wrist injuries.

- Do exercises that strengthen your hand and arm muscles.
- Stop, change, or take a break from activities that cause your symptoms.
- Reduce the speed and force of repetitive movements in activities such as hammering, typing, knitting, quilting, sweeping, raking, playing racquet sports, or rowing.
- Change positions when holding objects, such as a book or playing cards, for any length of time.
- Use your whole hand to grasp an object. Gripping with only your thumb and index finger can stress your wrist.
- Consider wearing gloves that support the wrist and have vibration-absorbing padding when working with tools that vibrate.
- Use safety measures, such as gloves, and follow instructions for the proper use of hand and power tools.
- Use caution when using knives in preparing food or craft activities. Supervise a child using knives or sharp scissors in craft activities.
- Wear protective gear, such as wrist guards, in sports activities.
- Review your work posture and body mechanics.
- Organize your work so that you can change your

position occasionally while maintaining a comfortable posture.

- Position your work so you do not have to turn excessively to either side.
- Keep your shoulders relaxed when your arms are hanging by your sides.
- When using a keyboard, keep your forearms parallel to the floor or slightly lowered and keep your fingers lower than your wrists. Allow your arms and hands to move freely. Take frequent breaks to stretch your fingers, hands, wrist, shoulders, and neck. If you use a wrist pad during breaks from typing, it's best to rest your palm or the heel of your hand on the support, rather than your wrist.

Reduce Falls

- Take steps to prevent falls and injuries in adults, such as removing any obstacles from your walking path.
- Take steps to prevent falls and injuries in babies and toddlers, such as not leaving your baby unattended in any infant seat or "sitting" toy.

General Prevention Tips

- Wear your seat belt in a motor vehicle.
- Don't carry objects that are too heavy.
- Use a step stool. Do not stand on chairs or other unsteady objects.
- Wear protective gear during sports or recreational activities, such as roller-skating or soccer. Supportive splints, such as wrist guards, may reduce your risk for injury.
- Warm up well and stretch before any activity. Stretch after exercise to keep hot muscles from

shortening and cramping.

- Use the correct techniques (movements) or positions during activities so that you do not strain your muscles.

- Avoid overusing your hand and wrist doing repeated movements that can injure your bursa or tendon. In daily routines or hobbies, examine activities in which you make repeated arm movements.

- Consider taking lessons to learn the proper techniques for sports. Have a trainer or person who is familiar with sports equipment check your equipment to see if it is well-suited for your level of ability, body size, and body strength.

- If you feel that certain activities at your workplace are causing pain or soreness from overuse, talk to your human resources department for information on alternative ways of doing your job or to discuss equipment modifications or other job assignments.

Keep Your Bones Strong

- Eat a nutritious diet with enough calcium and vitamin D, which helps your body absorb calcium. Calcium is found in dairy products, such as milk, cheese, and yogurt; dark green, leafy vegetables, such as broccoli; and other foods.

- Exercise and stay active. It is best to do weight-bearing exercise (walking, jogging, stair climbing, dancing, or lifting weights) for 45 to 60 minutes at least 4 days a week. Weight-bearing exercises stimulate new bone growth by working the muscles and bones against gravity. Exercises that are not weight-bearing, such as swimming, are good for your general health but do not stimulate new bone growth. Talk to your doctor about an exercise program that is right for you. Begin slowly, especially if you have been inactive. For more information, see the topic Fitness.

- Don't drink more than 2 alcoholic drinks a day if you are a man, or 1 alcoholic drink a day if you are a woman. People who drink more than this may be at higher risk for weakening bones (osteoporosis). Alcohol use also increases your risk of falling and breaking a bone.

- Do not smoke or use other tobacco products. Smoking puts you at a much higher risk of developing osteoporosis. It also interferes with blood supply and healing. For more information, see the topic Quitting Tobacco Use.

Jammed Finger

A jammed finger is a frustrating sports injury. It can happen in just about any sport, and while seemingly simple, can really put a damper on your ability to play. Learn more about finger sprains, how they happen, and what to do about them below.

What is a Jammed Finger?

A jammed finger, in medical terms, is a sprain of the joint capsule of the inter-phalangeal joints. What? In English? It is injury to the knuckles.

A joint sprain involves injury to ligaments or the joint capsule. Every joint in the body is comprised of both ligaments and joint capsule in order to connect the bones together. The fingers, although often overlooked, are no different. Just like other joints, the capsule and ligaments can be damaged if subjected to significant force...which leads us to how a jammed finger happens...

Jamming Your Finger

It has probably happended to you before. You were reaching out to catch the basketball, and it moved funny, or you weren't quite ready, and it caught you right on the end of your finger. It hurts like crazy, and kinda stuns you for a minute. That is how you jam your finger.

The force that hits the end of the finger is translated through the bones into the joint. Often, the ends of the phalanges (finger bones) are bruised at the knuckle, and this is what causes the swelling, as well as damage to the capsule.

There are other ways to suffer a finger sprain. You can get it bent the wrong way, or too far another way. You can get it stepped on, smashed between two helmets, hit with a baseball, or any other numerous ways that produce enough force to cause injury. Fingers are in the middle of most sports, and they tend to get hurt.

Symptoms of a Jammed Finger

Pain, swelling, loss of motion, and loss of strength are all very common symptoms of a jammed finger. Swelling within the joint is very obvious, and you can usually tell very easily when you have suffered a finger sprain.

One knuckle will swell up, and it will look noticibly bigger than the others. Unfortunately, this swelling often lasts for weeks if not months. Sometimes it never completely goes away.

Pain and motion usually come back fairly quickly, depending on how severe the sprain is.

Treating a Jammed Finger

Treating pain and swelling are the first steps of treating a jammed finger. As soon after injury as you can, use the R.I.C.E. Principles to help reduce your pain and discomfort. Depending on how much pain, swelling, and loss of motion you have, you may need to see your physician.

This is especially true if you took a pretty hard hit to the finger, or if it was bent backwards violently. You may have suffered a finger fracture and not just a sprain. It is sometimes hard to differentiate between the two, so an X-ray may be a good idea to be safe.

Once a fracture is ruled out, you can begin working on improving your range of motion and strength. Use ice and rest for a few days, and then begin trying to bend and straighten the finger. Do this gently, only pushing into mild discomfort. Gradually, your motion will return, as swelling goes down.

Some finger sprains may need to be splinted. If you have significant swelling and pain, see your physician, and they will direct you with treatment.

Conclusion

Jammed fingers are very common in sports, and they are ofen overlooked as insignificant. This is sometimes true, but a little rest and ice can go a long way to reduce the time it takes to heal, and to get things back to normal.

Don't assume that you just sprained your finger. If you have lots of swelling and pain, see your physician for an X-ray. Fingers, although overlooked, are extremely important to your sports participation, and in the rest of life.

11

CARE AND PREVENTION OF SPINE INJURIES

Severe spinal injury is infrequent during recreational or sporting activities compared to its incidence in high-velocity motor vehicle accidents. For example, only 4 head and neck injury fatalities in football occurred in 100,000 participants in 1968. Nevertheless, significant spinal injury does occur in contact and high-velocity sports. Spine injuries due to sports accounted for 14% of 1,447 cases in a series reported by Reid and Saboe and for 10% of injuries in children in study by Anderson and Schutt. The incidence of neurologic deficit and the location of injuries vary with the type of activity. In sports such as diving, rugby, snowmobiling, skiing and ice hockey, however, the incidence of neurologic deficit is high. Reid and Saboe reported a 67% incidence of paralysis due to cervical spine fractures in hockey players. Less significant lower spinal injury is more common with jumping, running, or dancing. Review of the essential osseous and ligamentous anatomy is crucial for proper interpretation and utilization of imaging techniques.

Osteology

The vertebral column is composed of 7 cervical, 12 thoracic, 5 lumbar, 5 sacral, and 4 cocygeal segments. The lateral masses of C-1 articulate with the occipital condyles at the base of the skull. The sacrum articulates with the innominate bones of the pelvis.

The typical vertebral body consists of the anterior body and the vertebral arch, which is composed of two pedicles and two paired laminae. The laminae join posteriorly to form the spinous process. In addition, there are transverse processes bilaterally. Four extensions from the lamina-pedicle junction form the apophyseal or facet joints. The facets articulate with the vertebre above and below. These apophyseal joints play an important role in determining the range and direction of motion of the vertebral column. Most of the weight-bearing function is provided by the vertebral bodies and interposed elastic vertebral discs. The apophyseal joints are also involved in weight-bearing, however, especially when one changes from the sitting to the standing position.

There are several anatomic features that distinguish the regions of the spine. The bodies of the cervical and lumbar vertebrae are wider in transverse than in anteroposterior diameter. The thoracic vertebral body is more uniform in AP and lateral diameter. In the upper thoracic region the vertebral bodies are somewhat heart shaped. The spinal canal in the cervical and lumbar region is triangular compared with the smaller, circular configuration in the thoracic region. The transverse processes in the cervical region contain anterior and posterior tubercles as well as a distinguishing feature, the foramen transversarium. The vertebral artery traverse this foramen from C-7 to C-1. The transverse processes in the thoracic region are directed dorsally, and T-1 through T-10 contain facets for rib articulation. Transverse processes in the lumber region project almost straight laterally and increase in sie from L-1 to L-3. The L-4 transverse process is shorter and directed more cephalad. The transverse process of L-5 is broader and sturdier and also is directed dorsally.

Spinous processes are short and often bifid in the cervical spine. The spinous process of C-7 is the longest and most prominent, whereas the spinous process of C-2 is short and bulbous. Spinous processes in the thoracic region are directed sharply caudate; they are long and narrow compared with the broad-based, short spinous processes in the lumbar region.

The articular facets differ significantly in the cervical, thoracic, and lumbar regions. In the cervical spine the articular facets angle approximately 20° in a caudad direction with the facet directed posteriorly. A similar but steeper angle is present in the thoracic region, and the facets are angled slightly dorsolterally. The facet joints in the lumbar region change abruptly, with the superior facets being directed dorsally and medially and the inferior facets being directed ventrally and laterlly. This results in restricted rotation in the lumbar region.

Cervical Vertebrae

The distinguishing feature of the cervical vertebrae is the formaen transversarium. In addition, there are several significant anatomic differences between C-1, C-2, C-7, and the remaining cervical vertebrae. The atlas has no vertebral body and lacks a true spinous process. C-1 is a ringlike structure with a large vertebral formaen bounded by the anterior and posterior arches. There are two large lateral masses that contain a superior articular facet. This facet articulates superiorly and medially with the occipital condyle. The inferior facet is directed medially and articulates with the superior facet of C-2. Medial to the lateral masses are tubercles for the attachment of the strong transverse ligament. The transverse processes of C-1 are also much larger compared with those of the remaining cervical vertebrae.

The C-2 vertebra has several distinguishing features. These include a prominent but short spinous process that is helpful in differentiating the level of the upper cervical spine when the entire spine is not included on a radiographic film. The odontoid or dens projects superiorly form the body of C-2 and articulates with the anterior ring of C-1. The spinal canal at C-2 is significantly smaller and rounder than that of C-1. The articular facets of C-2 are also atypical compared with those of the remaining cervical spine. The superior facets are directed in a superolateral direction at an angle of approximately 20°.

The C-3 through C-6 vertebrae are typical cervical vertebrae with triangular vertebral formain, and typically the facet joints are directed inferiorly at approximately 20°. C-7 can be distinguished by its prominent spinous process.

Thoracic Vertebrae

The upper and lower thoracic vertebrae have some features similar to those of the cervical or lumbar vertebrae. Thus the middle four thoracic vertebral bodies are most typical. In the upper thoracic spine the vertebral bodies are more triangular or heart shaped, with the apex of the triangle being directed ventrally. The vertebral bodies in the thoracic spine are typically target in AP than in transverse diameter. The thoracic vertebral body is 1.5 to 2.0 mm shorter ventrally than dorsally. This normal feature should not be confused with a compression fracture. Costal facets for rib articulations are a distinguishing feature of thoracic vertebrae. These are located on the inferior of ventral surface of the transverse process from T-1 to T-10 and at the junction of the body and pedicle from T-1 to T-

12. The last two ribs do not typically articulate with the transverse processes. The pedicles in the thoracic spine are short and thin, and the vertebral formaina are smaller and more circular than those in either the cervical or lumbar region. The transverse processes typically decrease in length as one progresses from T-1 to T-12. Orientation of the facets in the thoracic region is almost vertical. They are directed posteriorly and slightly laterally throughout the thoracic spine except at the T-12 level. Here the inferior facets face laterally to articulate with the superior facets of L-1.

Lumbar Vertebrae

The lambar vertebral bodies are larger than the thoracic vertebrae and typically are kidney shaped, with the transverse diameter being greater than the AP diameter. The vertical dimension of L-5 is greater anteriorly than posteriorly. As in the case of the cervical spine, the spinalcanal or the vertebral foramen is triangular in the lumbar region. The laminae in the lumbar region are strong and often symmetric. The pedicles are short and thick. The apophyseal joints arise from the lamina-pedicle junction. The superior facets are directed posteriorly and laterally. The laumbar vertebrae have no costal facets and no formina transversaria. The transverse processes of the first three lumbar vertebrae are straight and project almost dircctly laterally, increasing in length from L-1 through L-3. At L-4 and L-5 the transverse processes are shorter, with the transverse process of L-4 being directed somewhat dorsally and superiorly compared with the short, stout transverse process of L-5 .

Sacrum

In adults the sacrum is composed of five nonmovable segments. The discs are ossified and fused. The first sacral segment and C-1 are the only vertebrae with true lateral masses. The sacrum articulates with the ilia, forming paired synovial sacroiliac joints. Superiorly, two facets articulate with the inferior facets of L-5. Of the five sacral segments, the first is the largest. The size of the segments diminishes as one progresses inferiorly. The costal elements and transverse processes are fused. On the AP or formal view the ventral sacral foramina can be clearly visualized.

Ligamentous Anatomy

The fibrocartilaginous intervertebral discs are the main connecting segments between the vertebral bodies from C-2 through the sacrum. There may be rudimentary discs at the sacral levels, but the sacral segments are usually completely fused.

The nucleus pulposusn and anulus fibrosus are derived from the notochord embryologically. The discs, composed of the nucleus pulposus and anulus, contribute approximately one fourth to one-third of the height of the vertebral column. The configuration of the disc varies somewhat, depending upon the region of the vertebral column in which it is located. In the cervical region the discs are taller ventrally than dorsally. A similar situation is present in the lumbar region, In the thoracic region the discs are approximately equal in height anteriorly and posteriorly. The thickness of the disc in the lumbar region increases slightly as one progresses from L-1 to L-4, with the disc at the L-4 level being the largest. The L5-S1 disc is triangular and much thicker ventrally. The fibres of the anulus fibrosus develop in concentric rings running obliquely, with the superficial fibres blending into the anterior and posterior longitudinal ligaments.

The anterior longitudinal ligament is stronger and wider than the posterior longitudinal ligament. It is narrowest at its origin at the base of the skull and gradually widens to the level of its insertion on the pelvic surface of the sacrum.

The posterior longitudinal ligament lies within the vertebral foramen along the posterior surface of the vertebral body. This ligament is contiguous with the tectorial membrane superiorly and extends caudally into the sacral canal. The posterior longitudinal ligament blends with the fibres of the anulus fibrosus but is separated from the vertebral body by a venous plexus.

The ligamentum flavum is an elastic, thick, paired ligament that extends between the laminae of adjacent vertebrae. The ligaments blend with the articular capsules of the apophyseal joints. Posterior to the ligamentum flavum is the thinner intraspinous ligament, which joins the spinous processes and blends superficially with the supraspinous ligament. The supraspinous ligament in the cervical region is stronger and is called the ligamentum nuchae. This structure extends from the external occipital protuberance to the spinous process of C-7. Extending between the transverse processes are the intertransverse ligaments, which are best developed in the thoracic and lumbar regions and essentially are nonexistent in the cervical region. Also, in the cervical region the interspinous ligament may be sparse and disappear with age; thus if this ligament were torn secondary to trauma the significance of the injury would be questionable.

The apophyseal or facet joints are synovial joints with a fibrous capsule. Internally there are menisuslike tabs composed primarily of synovium and fatty tissue that project from the capsule into the joints. The articular capsules are more lax in the cervical spine, allowing more motion than in the remainder of the spine.

The ligamentous anatomy in the atlantoaxial region is more complex, requiring more emphasis. The posterior longitudinal ligament is continuous with the tectorial membrane that extends cephalad to the inner aspect of the foramen magnum. The transverse ligament lies ventral to the tectorial membrane. It is strong fibrous band that connects the tubercles of the lateral masses of C-1 posteriorly and maintains the relationship of the odontoid to the anterior ring of C-1. There are synovial joints between the odontoid and anterior ring at C-1 and between the odontoid and the transverse ligament. In addition, there are three ligaments extending vertically from the tip of the odonotoid. The apical ligament extends superiorly and attaches to the occipital bone. The two alar of check ligaments extend from the apex of the odontoid in a dorsilateral direction. The accessory ligament is a significant structure attaching at the base of the odontoid on either side. It is through this ligament that the odontoid receives part of its blood supply.

Neuroanatomy

The spinal cord with its meninges envelope lies within the vertebral foramen and extends in the adult form the foramenmagnum to the upper border of L-2. The vertebral foramen is bordered by the body anteriorly, the pedicles laterally, and the lamina posteriorly. The size of the vertebral foramen is largest in the lumbar and cervical regions, which coincides with the nerve distribution to the upper and lower extremities. The spinal cord occupies approximately 50% of the vertebral foramen. The remainder of the space is occupied by a the epidural venous plexus, which is intermixed with fat, connective tissue, and the protective meningeal portions of the spinal cord. The dura is a dense fibrous tube contiguous with the foramen magnum that extends to the level of the third sacralsegment. The dural sleeves surround each set of spinal nerve roots as they exit the dural sac. The pia mater is the thin innermost layer of the meninges that is applied to the spinal cord and nerve roots as they cross the subarachnoid space. More peripheral to the pia mater is the arachnoid, which encloses the subarachnoid space. The arachnoid, pia, and dura are united by the dentate ligaments that pass from the spinal cord to the dura. In the adult the spinal cord proper terminates at the conus medullaris. The filum terminale continues caudally until it blends with the posterior ligament and sacral canal. Both structure are enveloped in the dural sac to the S-2 level.

There are 31 pair of spinal nerves: 8 cervical, 12 thoracic, 5 lumbar, 5 scaral, and 1 coccygeal. Cervical nerve roots exit above the level of the adjacent vertebral body. In the remainder of the spine the nerve roots exist below the adjacent bodies.

CERVICAL SPINE TRAUMA

Cervical spine fractures, fracture-dislocations, and soft tissue injuries are less common in sports than in high-velocity motor vehicle accidents. Even so, up to 14% of adult and 10% of childhood cervical spine injuries are related to sports injuries. Common winter sports associated with cervical spine trauma include snowmobiling, skiing, tobogganing, and ice hockey. Other sports implicated in cervical spine trauma include football rugby, gymnastics, trampolining, and diving.

Mechanisms of Injury

Understanding the mechanisms of injury and the

structures, both bone and soft tissue, that may be affected is essential for proper selection of imaging techniques. The type and severity of cervical spine injury vary with the sport and mechanism of injury. The literature has provided numerous in-depth discussions of mechanisms of cervical spine injury.

Although most of the reports do not deal with sports injuries specifically, the mechanisms described can also frequently be applied to sports injuries.

The mechanism of injury is rarely pure. In one series of 420 cervical spine fractures and fracture-dislocations, most injuries could be classified into four groups. Hyperextension occurred in 38% of patients. Hyperflexion injuries were somewhat more common. Most were flexion-compression or disruptive hyperflexion injuries. This group included 12% of the total subjects in the series who had unilateral facet locking or perching. Vertical compression injuries occurred in 4% of the 420 patients. Radiographic classification could not be accomplished in 10% to 12% of the cases. These patients presented with radiographic findings that did not allow exact determination of the mechanism of injury. These injuries included nondisplaced odontoid fractures, in which the radiographic features were insufficient to determine the mechanism of injury even when combined with clinical data. Spinous process fractures may result from flexion, extension, or direct trauma. If there are no associated fractures, classification is difficult in such cases as well.

Dafner and colleagues describe similar findings in 646 cervical spine injuries. Radiographic features allowed identification of four basic mechanisms of injury in the majority of patients.

Hyperflexion Injuries

There are many descriptive terms in the literature that attempt to define the motion of the cervical spine and the direction of the force that result is injury. Certain of these terms are extremely helpful, and others are confusing. Flexion injuries have been classified a disruptive compressive, and shearing in nature. Disruptive hyperflexion indicates that the blow was directed upward toward the occipital region, resulting in forward flexion of the head. The major force is applied to the posterior ligaments and spinous processes, resulting in distraction of the spinous processes. If the force is sufficient and the motion of the head continues, the posterior ligaments are interrupted, resulting in an unstable injury. The cervical spine may then return to a nearly normal position, dispending upon the extent of force applied. In this case, the lateral radiograph may demonstrate hyphosis with widening of the interspinous distance and facet joints. If the disruptive force continues, however, unilateral or bilateral locking of the facets occurs, depending on the degree of associated rotation. Some authorities prefer to consider unilateral locking a flexion-rotation injury. As mentioned earlicr, this type of injury occurred in 12% of 420 patients in one series. Flexion-frotation injuries may be subtle, with only minimal anterior subluxation. On the lateral vicw the facet joints at the level of thc injury rotate, giving a bow-tie appearance. Oblique views will usually demonstrate the injury more clearly.

Compressive hyperflexion injuries occur when a force is applied to the top of the head, resulting in forward arching of the head. These injuries are common in contact sports. The main force is distributed along the vertebral bodies. As described earlier, the force is mainly compressive, and thus the posterior ligaments may remain intact. Wedge fractures of the bodies, teardrop fractures, and fracture-dislocations may result.

Harris states that the flexion teardrop injury is the most unstable lesion of all. In this situation the vertebrae above the injury move anterorly and the vertebrae below posteriorly in a circular direction.

Compressive shearing forces result from a force directed to the back of the head with the head moving forward. The end result may be an anteriorly displaced fracture of the odontoid. Atlantoaxial and atlantooccipital dislocations are rare but may also occur in this type of injury. This injury is unusual even in contact sports.

Hyperextension Injuries

Hyperextension injuries may occur when a force is applied to the mandible in an upward direction, leading to distruption of the anterior longitudinal ligament and disc. The lateral radiograph may be normal or reveal soft tissue swelling with displacement of the prevertebral fat stripe. Widening of the anterior disc space may also be evident. A small chip fracture, usually from the anteroinferior aspect of the vertebral body, may be noted. The radiographic changes may be very subtle, and further confusion may be added by the presence of significant neurologic deficits. Neurologic damage often is the result of AP compression of the cord, leading to a decrease in the AP diameter of the spinal canal and vascular compromise of the cord. Infolding of the ligamentum flavum may also play a part in the cord impingement.

Hyperextension may also result from blows directed to the vertex of the skull, when most of the force is absorbed by the posterior arch. Fractures of the spinous process, lamina, pedicles, and articular pillars may result. Anterior subluxation may occur, which on the lateral radiogrph could be mistaken for a flexion injury. Oblique and pillar views will demonstrate the posterior arch fractures and aid in differentiating the mechanism of injury. In these cases, conventional tomography or computed tomography is often needed to evaluate the neural arch. Facial injuries are also common in patients with hyperextension injuries. Finally, anterior shearing forces result in posterior fracture dislocations in the upper cervical spine.

Vertical Compression (Axial Loading) Injuries

Pure vertical compression or axial ioading may result in a typical Jefferson fracture or a burst fracture in the lower cervical spine. The spin must be in a nearly neutral position when the vertical force is applied. Although axial loading injuries are common in contact sports, some degree of flexion, extension, or rotation is typically present as well. Usually there is an asymmetric vertical compression with lateral flexion. This may result in a compression fracture of one of the lateral masses of C-1, a pillar fracture, or a stinger. Fractures of the uncinate process of a transverse process fracture may also occur. Axial forces with flexion may also lead to lower cervical burst fractures.

Minor Injuries

Most sports injuries are due to minor sprains or strains from hyperflexion, hyperextension, or rotary forces. Complete disruption of a muscle or ligament without associated fracture is unusual but can occur. This can lead to an unstable injury with subtle radiographic findings. Motion studies or magnetic resonance imaging may be required for detection and classification of these injuries.

The so-called stinger usually results from lateral flexion but can also occur with flexion and extension injuries. Sudden lateral flexion during tackling or blocking in football is often described. The injury result in traction or impingement of nerves of the brachial plexus, leading to pain, numbness, and tingling that extend down the arm on the involved side. The C5-6 levels are most commonly involved. Usually the symptoms clear in several minutes. With significant or repeated episodes, however, the symptoms may be more severe.

Three grades of stinger injury have been described. Athletes with grade I injuries recover in a few minutes. Grade 2 injuries lead to decreased strength in the deltoid, infraspinatus, supraspinatus, and biceps muscles that may last up to 3 weeks. With grade 3 injuries the motor and sensory deficits may last 1 year or more. Electromyographic abnormalities may be evident with grade 2 and 3 injuries. Radiographic findings are unusual, however, except in severe or recurrent injuries. In this setting, disc space narrowing or subtle fractures may be noted in up to 25% of cases.

Avulsion injuries are generally stable and do not necessarily require withdrawal from contact sports once they have healed. These injuries are most common with hyperextension or hyperflexion. Clay shoveler's fractures and anteroinferior C-2 body avulsion occur most frequently.

Traumatic disc herniations are uncommon but may lead to neurologic symptoms. Herniated cervical discs may present with pain, reduced motion, and sensory changes in the upper extremities. Loss of reflexes in the distribution of the affected nerve root may be noted on physical examination. MRI or CT myelography may be needed if conservative therapy fails.

Imaging of Cervical Spine Injuries

Acutely injured patients with suspected spinal trauma must be properly immobilized until the radiographic examination is complete and treatment is instituted. Radiographic evaluation can be accomplished only when close communication between the radiologist and clinicians is maintained. A well-organized approach will ensure optimal use of routine films, tomography, CT, MRI, and other techniques in determining the extent of injury and stability of the lesion.

A simple radiographic table with an overhead tube capable of big positioned at different angles is sufficient for evaluation of the spine. The necessary views for evaluation of the cervical, thoracic, and lumbar spine can be obtained easily. We utilize a C-arm Versigraph, which allows AP, lateral, and oblique views without moving the patient. In addition, tomograms can be obtained in the AP, lateral, oblique, and transaxial projections. Conventional radiographic equipment would require the patient to be placed in the oblique or lateral position to obtain tomograms in these projections.

Routine Radiography of the Cervical Spine

Routine radiographs remain the most effective screening technique for evaluating spinal trauma. Radio graphic evaluation of the cervical spine should be thoroughly and completely monitored by the rediologist until the degree of injury has been established. Such an evaluation demands that the examination be tailored to the patient's clinical symptoms. The initial evaluation should include lateral, oblique, AP, and odontoid views. Pillar views may also be indicated. The head must be turned for pillar views, however; therefore, the other views should be studied first to determine whether it id safe or necessary to move the head for pillar views.

Lateral View

The lateral view is the most important radiographic view. Ninety per cent of the significant pathology can be detected on the lateral view.

There are many features that should be carefully examined on the lateral view. It is essential that all seven cervical vertebrae be well demonstrated. Ideally T-1 should also be visible on the lateral view. The lateral view allows assessment of the following structures: the anterior and posterior arches of C-1, the odonioid, vertebral bodies, disc spaces, facet joints, and spinous processes. The lateral radiograph shows that the body of T-1 is larger than that of C-7, which can give the false impression of subluxation. This fact must be kept in mind when evaluating patients with flexion injuries.

Careful attention should also be paid to the soft tissues in the prevertebral space. In the adult the measurement of the soft tissue from the anterioinferior margin of C-2 to the retropharyngeal wall should not exceed 7 mm. The distance from the posterior wall of the trachea to the anteroinferior margin of C-6 should not exceed 14 mm in children and 22 mm in adults. Care must be taken in measuring this distance in young people and children because changes on inspiration can simulate swelling. Nasogastric and endotracheal tubes invalidate measurements of the retropharyngeal space. The posterior portions of the maxillary antra and mandible may also provide a clue to the mechanism of injury. These structures can be partially studied on most lateral views of the cervical spine. Mandibular fractures are often associated with hyperextension injuries.

Odontoid View

The odontoid view is obtained with the patient's mouth open as wide as possible. The beam is centered over the open mouth and aligned perpendicularly to the cassette. The neck should not be extended or the posterior occiput may obscure the odontoid. This view allows on to study the odontoid, lateral masses, and transverse processes of C-1 If the patient and tube are properly aligned, the spinous process of C-2 will be midline. Spaces between the teeth and the inferior margin of the posterior arch of C-1 may overlap the odontoid and should not be confused with fractures. It the odontoid is not well demonstrated, the tube can be angled to reduce bony overlap.

Oblique Views

The oblique views after acute trauma are obtained by angling the C-arm 45° from the horizontal. In the upright position the patient is rotated, so that the side away from the film is demonstrated. Detail is improved on the Versigraph. Also, magnification caused by the distance between the patient and the film may assist in detecting subtle fractures. With a conventional table, oblique views are obtained by angling the tube 35° to 40° to the horizontal with a 15° cranial angle. The oblique views provide excellent detail of the uncinate processes, pedicles, laminae, and alignment of facet joints. These views are particularly important in detecting facet subluxations and dislocations.

Pillar Views

A significant number of cervical spine fractures involve the posterior arch. Pillar views are useful in evaluation of the articular pillars and laminae. This view is obtained by angling the tube 25° to 30° toward the feet and can be performed with the patient's neck extended or rotated 45°. The AP, lateral, and oblique views must be reviewed first to be certain that there is no unstable or significant injury. Rotation of the head or extension of the neck should be avoided if a significant injuries evident on initial views. Pillar fractures, if present, are almost always stable but can result in significant pain and radiculopathy.

Obtaining high-quality pillar views can be difficult. Conventional tomography or CT is more frequently utilized in our practice.

Flexion and Extension views

Flexion and extension views of the cervical spine are performed to evaluate stability. The examination is most often indicated to exclude ligament instability after trauma or to determine whether fractures are healed and stable. This examination should be performed fluoroscopically so that a true lateral position can be properly attained and the degree of motion monitored. Some clinicians perform upright lateral views before clearing patients with otherwise normal cervical spine series.

The patient should sit or stand. Physiologic extension and flexion in the lateral position are monitored fluoroscopically. The extension manoeuvre is performed initially, and alignment of the vertebrae and anterior ligament structures are studied. The patient is then asked to flex the cervical spine slowly so that alignment, subluxation, facet joint widening, and spinous process motion can be carefully observed. The criteria discussed in routine evaluation of the lateral cervical spine can be applied. Subtle changes may be important, however, and care must be taken not to overlook posterior ligament damage. Vertebral body subluxation in flexion should not exceed 1 mm.

Conventional and Computed Tomography

Tomographic techniques are often helpful

indetermining the full extent of injury. CT is most frequently selected, but conventional tomogrpahy is preferred in patients with suspected odontoid fractures or when the fracture line may be parallel to the CT image plane. In this setting, fractures may be overlooked because of partial volume effects.

The choice of examination is based on several factors, including patient status, type of injury suspected, and equipment availability. Most skeletal tomography is performed with complex motion techniques as opposed to linear tomography. This would reure moving the patient. The C-arm unit permits linear tomography in the AP, lateral, oblique, and axial planes without moving the patient. We routinely obtain AP and lateral tomograms. Tomography is most useful for evaluating odontoid fractures, fractures in the plane of CT imaging, and fractures of the facet joints and for demonstrating contiguous segments.

CT is most useful for evaluating patients with neurologic deficits, detecting bone fragments in the spinal canal or neural foraminal, and preoperative planning of complex injuries. On occasion, intrathecal contrast medium plus CT used to evaluate dural tears and nerve root injuries. Nonionic water-soluble contrast medium can be injected via the lumbar route or by C1-C2 puncture. In most patients 5-mm contiguous slices are adequate for evaluating spinal fractures. If reconstruction in the coronla and sagittal planes or three-dimensional processing is required, much thinner slices should be obtained. Three-millimetre slices at 2-mm intervals or 1.5-mm contiguous slices provide superior reconstructed images.

Magnetic Resonance Imaging

MRI is an established technique for evaluating the

musculoskeletal system. Soft tissue contrast is superior to that obtained with CT, and images can be obtained in the axial, coronal, oblique, and sagittal planes. Fine bone detail is not as well demonstrated with MRI compared to CT. Also, the confining nature of the MR gantry reduces patient access, especially on high-field imagers. Therefore, MRI is not as frequently utilized in the acutely injured patient with multiple trauma.

MRI techniques have improved significantly over the past several years. Although there are numerous sequences from which to choose, most clinicians utilize both T1- and T2-weighted images to evaluate completely the osseous and soft tissue anatomy. Sagittal T1-weighted images provide a good screening technique for changes in the vertebral body. T2-Weighted images are more useful for evaluation of the spinal cord and discs. Muscle tears and ligament injuries should also be more easily appreciated on T2-weighted images. Spin-echo T2-weighted images require 9 to 16 minutes of imaging time. New gradient-echo techniques with reduced flip angles can provide images with T2-weighting in about 4 minutes, which is advantageous in patients with spinal cord injury. The use of gadolinium DTPA with T1-weighted images is also helpful for more complete evaluation of the spinal cord.

To date, MRI has been most useful for evaluation of the spinal cord and discs. Kulkarni et al described patterns of cord abnormality that are useful in predicting neurologic recovery. The potential for evaluating posterior muscle and ligament injury also exists, but result are preliminary at the time. Currently, MRI is most often used for evaluating patients with cord injury in the acute and chronic setting.

Major Cervical Spine Injuries

The anatomic relationships of the upper cervical spine are unique, and the mechanisms of injury differ somewhat from those affecting the lower cervical spine. Therefore, in discussing specific cervical spine injuries the upper and lower segments are presented separately. As with injuries incurred in motor vehicle accidents, most sport-related injuries in adults involve the lower cervical spine. In children up to 25% of injuries occur above C-4.

Upper Cervical Spine

Injuries involving the occipital condyles and atlanto occipital articulation are rare. Fractures of the condyle may result from shearing or rotary forces and blows to the calvarium from above, similar to the mechanism that result in a Jefferson fracture. These injuries may disrupt the hypoglossal canal, injuring the jugular vein and cranial nerves IX, X, and XI. Often, however, the trauma may seem minor with no neurologic deficit. As will other upper cervical spine injuries, tomography is extremely valuable. Routine radiographs are often normal, and CT may miss this fracture because of partial volume effects.

Atlantooccipital dislocations are also rare. This injury usually occurs in high-velocity motor vehicle accidents. Snowmobiling, auto racing, and tobogganing may also lead to this injury. At the Mayo Clinic we noted three atlantooccipital dislocations due to snowmobiling in 1 year. The lesion is usually the result of shearing forces directed either to the face or to the occipital region. Death due to brain stem injury typically follows this injury. Atlantooccipital dislocation is more common in children owing to their smaller condyles and the more horizontal articular relationship of the condyles with the lateral masses of the atlas.

Radiographically, the diagnosis is usually obvious on the lateral view of the skull or cervical spine. The occipital condyles lose their normal articular relationship with the atlas, and a large hematoma is present in the retropharyngeal space.

Atlas

In our experience fractures of the atlas account for approximately 4% of all spinal injuries. Other investigators report a similar incidence. These injuries, although due to adial forces, are infrequent in athletes. Five types of fractures have been described on the basis of the anatomic region affected: fractures of the anterior arch, posterior arch, lateral mass, and transverse process and the Jefferson fracture. Fractures most commonly involve the lateral masses and the posterior arch. Sherk and Nicholson reported that posterior arch fractures account for 67% of fractures of the atlas. Posterior arch fractures are the result of hyperextension injuries in which the arch is compressed between the occipital and spinous process of the axis. Associated injuries are common. In one study, spinous process fractures of C-7 were evident in 25% of patients with posterior arch fractures of C-1. Because posterior arch fractures are hyperextension injuries, one should not be surprised by the frequently associated facial injuries.

Pure Jefferson fractures result from a force directed vertically to the skull. The force is transmitted to the ocipital condyles, which leads to lateral displacement of the lateral masses of the atlas. The lateral displacement is a result of the anatomic configuration of these articulations. Fractures typically occur in the anterior and posterior arches. The anterior and, more specifically, the posterior arch are the weak points in the ring of the atlas. Less commonly, horizontal fractures of the anterior arch occur. This injury also results from hyperextension and avulsion at the insertion of the longus colli. It is essential to exclude other associated hyperextension injuries.

Neurologic complications with atlas fractures are rare. Significant retropharyngeal hemorrhage resulting in difficulty in breathing has been reported, however.

Radiographically, most injuries of C-1 can be detected on the AP odontoid view or on the lateral view of the cervical spine or skull. Several significant features noted on the AP odontoid view or AP tomograms should be stressed. Outward displacement of the lateral masses of the atlas of greater than 6.9 mm indicates a tear or avulsion of the transverse ligament. Normal features, however, such as the insertion of the transverse ligament and bipartite superior facets should not be confused with fractures. Subtle changes may require conventional tomography or CT for complete evaluation. CT is especially useful in evaluating the ring of the atlas.

Posterior and rotary dislocations are uncommon and occur more frequently in children and young adults as a result of rotation of the head, which may occur in wrestling or tackling with the arms about the head. Rotary dislocation requires 45° of rotation of C-1 on the axis for locking to occur. This condition differs from the rotary fixation described by Fielding and Hawkins. Sixty-five degrees of rotation is required for fixation to occur if the transverse ligament and odontioid are anatomically normal. If the ligament is interrupted, less rotation is required. Cord injury and vertebral artery injury have been reported with rotary fixation. Fielding and Hawkins defined the following four types of injuries:

- Type I: rotary fixation without anterior subluxation of the atlas on the axis.

• Type II: rotary fixation with 3 to 5 mm of atlantoaxial subluxation.

• Type III: rotary fixation with greater than 5 mm of atlantoaxial subluxation.

• Type IV: rotary fixation with posterior atlantoaxial subluxation

Type I is the most common lesion reported. The patient usually presents with the head rotated to the side. Neurologic deficits are rare. The exact etiology is unclear, but fixation may be related to capsular entrapment in the atlantoaxial facets.

Radiographically, the AP and lateral odonotoid views may be sufficient for diagnosis. CT is most accurate for evaluation, however, and allows differentiation from torticollis or simple rotation more radilly than routine radiographs.

Axis

Fractures of the odontiod and pedicles account for 80% of injuries to the axis. The vertebral body is for 80% of injuries to the axis. The vertebral body is involved in about 15% of cases, usually through the anteroinferior chip fracture. The facets, laminae, and spinous processes are less frequently involved.

Odontoid fractures may result from anterior shearing posterior shearing, or lateral flexion injuries. Obviously, these are most common in contact sports, snowmobiling, auto racing, and the like. Odonotoid fractures account for 11% to 13% of all cervical spine fractures. Patients with odonotoid fractures usually present with neck pain and rarely have neurologic symptoms. Even if there is displacement of the fractures, there is usually sufficient space to prevent cord injury.

In a significant number of cases, odonotoid fractures are undisplaced and subtle, requiring tomography for definitive diagnosis and classification. The mechanism of injury in these cases is often difficult to determine. If the fracture is slightly displaced, the mechanism of injury is more easily established. When the fracture is displaced, the lateral view of the skull or cervical spine and the open mouth odontoid view are usually adequate for diagnosis.

Radiographically, one should check carefully for retropharyngeal soft tissue swelling, which may be the only clue to an odontoid fracture. Tomography is frequently required for diagnosis and classification of the fractures. The classification system of Anderson and D'Alonzo is commonly utilized and is helpful in determining proper management and prognosis of the fracture. The classification divides odontoid fractures into three types: type I, oblique fracture of the tip of the odontoid; type II, fracture of the base of the odontoid; and type III, fracture entering the body of the axis.

A significant number of type II odonotoid fractures will be overlooked on routine radiographs. Also, CT may miss this injury because the fracture line may lie entirely within the image plane. Therefore, AP and lateral tomograms may be the best technique. Tomograms should be considered whenever symptoms are present even if routine views are normal. Both AP and lateral views are necessary because these injuries may be subtle.

Type III fractures account for about 33% of odonotoid fractures. These fractures are frequently impacted anteriorly, and anterior displacement can be identified in up to 90% of patients. Undisplaced type III fractures almost always unite with proper treatment. Neurologic involvement is slightly less common than with type II fractures. Nonunion is common if anterior displacement exceeds 5 mm.

Fractures of the neural arch of the axis result from hyperextension, and usually anterior subluxation of C-2 on C-3 is evident on the lateral radiograph. The lesion, as originally described, occurred as a result of judicial hanging. This mechanism of hyperextension and sustained distraction resulted in death. Flexion compression and flexion-distraction have also been implicated in hangman's fracture.

Although hangman's fractures have been considered pedicle fractures, this may be anatomically incorrect. Burke and Harris prefer the term traumatic spondylolisthesis of C-2 because by definition C-2 does not have true pedicles. This may be true, but the terminology with not change quickly; the term pedicle fracture will probably continue to be used.

Fractures of the body of the axis occurred in 13% to 15% of patients in the study by Burke and Harris. These fractures were all the result of hyperextension injuries and usually involved the anteroinferior margin of the vertebral body. Soft tissue swelling was common and often marked.

Isolated fractures of the lamina, spinous process, and facets of the axis are uncommon. Facet fractures of the axis are often associated with compression-rotation or lateral compression injuries, which result in associated lateral mass fractures of the atlas.

Lower Cervical Spine

In adults, injuries to the lower cervical spine occur four times more frequently than upper cervical spine fractures. Axial loading and flexion are the most common mechanisms of injury in athletes. Also, injuries at the C3-4 level tend to occur more commonly in sports injuries compared to motor vehicle accidents. The location of the fracture varies with the force or mechanism of injury.

Vertebral Arch Fractures

Fractures of the lamina are usually due to hyperextension injuries. Spinous process fractures are commonly associated with these fractures. Most laminar fractures occur in the C5-7 region. Pillar views and tomography are often necessary to detect laminar fractures. CT may also be helpful, but in the study several cases of undisplaced fractures not evident on CT were easily demonstrated with conventional tomography. This is true of any undisplaced fracture in which the fracture is aligned parallel to the slice. The increased utilization of tomography in our practice may be at least partially responsible for the higher incidence of laminar fractures in our series because of a higher rate of detection. Fractures of the lamina frequently extend into the base of the spinous process, resulting in a displaced spinous process. This should not be confused with the more benign clay shoveler's fracture. Laminar fractures with spinous process involvement have reported frequently with hyperextension injuries of the type V classification.

Pedicle fractures may be detected in up to 25% of vertebral arch injuries. Most pedicle fractures occur at C-2, but pedicle fractures are also noted in the lower cervical spine with hyperextension injuries. These injuries may be visible on lateral or oblique views. Conventional tomography or CT is frequently necessary for diagnosis. Acheson et al reported that 82% of pedicle fractures were overlooked on plain films but were detected with CT. Spinous process fractures account for 22% of vertebral arch injuries. Most spinous process fractures occur at the C5-T1 level. This fracture may result from direct trauma, hyperextension, or hyperflexion, and it is only through careful evaluation of the remaining vertebral units that the mechanism of injury may be established. On the AP view a double spinous process may be the only clue to an unsuspected spinous process fracture. In other cases the lateral view is usually most useful.

Fractures of the articular pillars have been reported to be the most common arch fracture. These injuries usually occur at the C-6 level. In one series pillar fractures occurred in 16% of vertebral arch fractures The mechanism of injury is usually hyperextension or lateral flexion. Occasionally, the AP view will demonstrate the lesion. These fractures are best demonstrated on pillar views or CT. Up to 60% will be overlooked on plain film examinations. There is usually no cord injury with a pillar fracture, but radiculopathy may result, especially if proper treatment is not instituted.

Facet fractures represented 9% of vertebral arch fractures in our study. These were most common with hyperflexion and flexion-rotation injuries. Oblique and lateral views may demonstrate this lesion, but conventional tomography or CT is usually required. Radicular symptoms are common with solitaly facet fractures. Facet fractures are usually detected with multiple injuries, including injuries of the posterior ligaments and disc.

Transverse process fractures are uncommon. The injury results from lateral flexion or direct trauma. Associated upper rib fractures are not uncommon.

Vertebral Body Fractures

Vertebral body fractures are common with sports injuries due to axial loading and flexion injuries. Most fractures are in the C5-7 region, but C3-4 lesions are also common in athletes. Fractures are usually evident on the AP and lateral views, with oblique views providing additional information. Tomography and CT are less frequently required for detection of vertebral body fractures, but evaluation of fragment position and classification is aided with CT.

Vertebral body fractures have several radiographic presentations: chip fractures, usually of the anterosuperior or anteroinferior margin; triangular fractures; burst fractures; wedge fractures, usually anterior but also lateral; uncinate process fractures; and sagittal fractures. Care must be taken not to mistake overlying structures for vertebral body fractures.

Chip fractures are commonly due to hyperflexion injuries and hyperextension injuries. After hyperextension injury, the fracture fragment is avulsed with the anterior lognitudinal ligament and in most instances enters the disc space. Hyperflexion injuries are often associated with posterior ligament disruption and are therefore unstable. Hyperextension injuries are usually stable unless the fracture of the body is associated with ap posterior arch fracture, in which case the lesion is unstable.

Larger triangular or teardrop fractures of the vertebral body are more significant. Most involve the anteroinferior body. The majority of triangular fractures involve the lower cervical spine. Neurologic involvement, usually quadriplegia, occurs in more than 80% of patients.

Simple compression fractures are most often anterior and result from flexion-compression injuries. The posterior ligaments may be intact, depending upon the degree of associated posterior element distraction.

The posterior ligaments must be evaluated at some point during treatment to be certain that the lesion is stable. This requires fluoroscopically controlled flexion and extension views.

Lateral wedge fractures and uncinate fractures are the result of asymmetric vertical compression or lateral flexion injuries.

Soft Tissue and Miscellaneous Injuries

Most significant ligament injuries involve the posterior complex. In one series 73% of these injuries occurred at the C5-7 level. Anterior ligament injuries are most common in the C2-4 and C6-7 intervals. Often the changes noted radiographically will aid in determining whether ligament injury has occurred. Posterior ligament injuries are unstable if complete disruption has occurred, and one must guard against overlooking the often subtle changes associated with this injury.

The same forces that result in isolated ligament disruption, if continued, may lead to unilateral or bilateral facet dislocation or locking. In athletes these injuries occur infrequently.

Anterior ligament injuries are often associated with anteroinferior chip fractures of the vertebral body. The mechanism of injury is disruptive hyperextension. These injuries are most common at the C2-4 and C6-7 levels. Changes may be subtle, with hematoma or displacement of the prevertebral fat stripe being the only indication of injury. Facial fractures and central cord syndrome are frequently present. MRI is useful in this setting.

Neural injury may be difficult to evaluate with imaging techniques. Brachial plexus injuries are most easily evaluated with MRI. Nerve root avulsion or contrusion has been evaluated with CT myelography and MRI.

THORACOLUMBAR SPINE TRAUMA

Anatomic differencesin the cervical, thoracic, and lumbar spine must be considered in any discussion of trauma to these regions. In the thoracic spine a slight kyphotic curve is normally present. This is in contrast to the lordotic curves evident in the cervical and lumbar regions. Also, the spinal canal in the thoracic region is circular and smaller in diameter than in the cervical or lumbar portions of the spine. As one progresses inferiorly, the vertebral bodies increase in size and the discs in height, resulting in an increasing resistance to vertical compression forces.

The lumbar segment is similar to the cervical segment in that both contain a greater potentioal for motion than the thoracic segment. The large paraspinal muscles in the lumbar region provide more stability than the cervical musculature, however. Owing to differences in range of motion, transition in the facet joints, and other anatomic factors, the thoracolumbar junction is the area most susceptible to injury. Thus the majority of injuries occur at this level.

Mechanisms of Injury

The majority of athletically related thoracolumbar injuries involve the paraspinal soft tissues. Strains and sprains occur most frequently. Stress injuries to the low back are also common, however, and have been noted in football players, cross-country skiers, and gymnasts. Horne et al reported progressive Scheuermann's disease and vertebral wedging in the thoracic spine in water ski jumpers due to repetitive compression forces.

The mechanisms of injury in the thoracolumbar

spine are similar to those in the cervical spine, but because of significant anatomic differences the results and presentation may vary.

Hyperflexion Injuries

Hyperflexion injuries are by far the most common injury in the thoracic and lumbar spine. Most often the injury is due to flexion-compression forces that result in a simple anterior wedge fracture of the vertebral body. The posterior complex is almost always intact; therefore, this is a stable injury.

The axis of the force in hyperflexion injuries is centered in the nucleus pulposus or in the midportion of the intervertebral disc. Thus the appearance of the injury may vary, depending upon the spinal level involved. In the upper thoracic region the discs are narrower, and the fracture is more typically a true anterior wedge fracture. In the thoracic region, especially the upper thoracic spine, the anterior height of the vertebral bodies is normally 1.5 mm less than the posterior height. In the lower thoracic and lumbar regions the discs are larger and more effective as shock absorbers. Thus herniation into the cartilaginous end plates is more likely to occur in the lower thoracic and lumbar regions.

The degree of compression and changes in the disc space are important in wedge fractures of the vertebral bodies. If compressions greater than 50% and if the disc space is narrowed, the prognosis is less favourable. These findings along with multiple contiguous wedge fractures may lead to delayed instability. Multiple contiguous wedge fractures in the upper thoracic region may lead to cord deficits.

Flexion-Rotation Injuries

Flexion-rotation injuries of the thoracolumber

spine are uncommon. When they occur, the are among the most unstable of spinal injuries. The injury usually occurs at the thoracolumbar junction owing to the transition in the facet joints. The incidence of neurologic deficits approaches 70%. This injury is easily overlooked because it is uncommon and, more important, because reduction of the dislocation tends to occur in the supine position.

Radiographic features of the injury are similar to those of a unilateral locked facet in the cervical spine. On the AP view the spinous process may be rotated to the side of the involvement, and a fracture through the upper endplate may be present. The disc space may appear asymmetric or tilted to one side. On the lateral view the disc space is often narrowed and the interspinous distance increased. A slice fracture of the upper vertebral body is usually more obvious on the lateral view. Fractures of the articular processes and lamiane frequently require tomography or CT for detection. CT is most useful in evaluating the degree of involvement of the spinal canal.

Vertical Compression Injuries

Vertical compression injuries result in burst fractures of the vertebral bodies with outward displacement of fracture fragments, herniation of the disc into the endplates, and posterior extension of the disc and fracture fragments into the spinal canal. Burst fractures are uncommon, accounting for only 1.5% of spinal injuries. Most injuries occur at the T12-L2 level. Although these injuries are potentially stable, the incidence of neurologic involvement is high owing to displacement of bone fragments into the spinal canal. Because at least tow columns are involved and it may be difficult to evaluate the posterior ligmant, these fractures should be considered unstable.

Burst fractures can usually be seen on the AP and lateral views. Such fractures invôlve multiple bony fragments and compression of the body and disc space. The interpedicular distance is increased on the AP view, and if tomograms are obtained arch fractures are also common. The posterior vertebral line is usually abnormal on the lateral view. Although the degree of spinal canal involvement can often be appreciated on the lateral view or lateral tomogram, CT is the technique of choice for evaluation of the spinal canal. Bony fragments, dural tears, and epidural hematomas may be detected with this modality.

Hyperextension Injuries

The majority of hyperextension injuries occur in the midlumbar region and are related to direct blows to the back. Lateral radiographs reveal posterior subluxation of the vertebral body above the level at which the trauma occurred. The incidence of neurologi injury in these patients is not significant, and healing may occur without resideual pain.

Radiographic findings with hyperextension injuries in the thoracolumbar spine are similar to those noted in the cervical spine. The features are best detected on the lateral view. The disc space may be widened anteriorly, and the posterior structures may be fractured as a result of compression forces. CT is useful in evaluation of the spinal canal and subtle fractures. Mild subluxation or position changes can be difficult to evaluate on axial images.

12

CARE AND PREVENTION OF HIP AND PELVIC INJURIES

INTRODUCTION

Hip pain in the young athlete can be a diagnostic and treatment dilemma for the clinician. In the past decade, progress in imaging and operative techniques have provided tools to better outfit the orthopedist involved in the care of these patients. Hip pain can be intra-articular or extra-articular, and it is important to distinguish between the two. The differential diagnosis for extra-articular hip pain includes apophyseal avulsion fractures, snapping iliotibial band over the greater trochanter, snapping hamstring over the ischial tuberosity, psoas snapping, psoas tendonitis, hip pointer, and even inguinal hernia. Intra-articular pathology includes all intracapsular sources of pain, including femoral neck stress fracture, ligamentum teres pathology, labral tears, chondral injuries, loose bodies, and slipped capital femoral epiphysis. The treating physician should be aware of pediatric conditions such as hip dysplasia and Legg–Calve Perthes disease, which can predispose the patient to hip pain as adolescents. Although many young patients may be treated with nonoperative means for their hip pain, the physician should be aware of new hip arthroscopic techniques that may be appropriate for their patients.

The runner is especially at risk for development of injury to the hip and pelvis secondary to chronic repetitive microtrauma. The key to treatment is establishing complete and accurate diagnosis, and, in particular, identifying the functional biomechanical deficits in the kinetic chain that contribute to this repetitive microtrauma. A long-term successful outcome and prevention of reinjury are more likely if the focus of rehabilitation is on the restoration of the functional kinetic chain, rather than on a specific injured tissue. For example, the typical treatment of "iliotibial band syndrome" is a stretching protocol that frequently is unsuccessful in the long-term improvement of symptoms. A functional biomechanical approach might identify that the injured runner has lack of calcaneal eversion and a structurally rigid supinated foot. These functional biomechanical deficits would lead to inadequate internal rotation of the tibia and femur and result in inhibition or decreased recruitment of the gluteal muscles, in particular the gluteus medius. Restoring pronation throughout the lower extremity would require joint play techniques or functional joint mobilizations for the foot and ankle. In addition, a running shoe with a cushioned heel may be necessary to promote pronation and to attenuate shock. Exercises that integrate foot and hip function, including balance reaches, lunges and step-downs, are prescribed to stimulate the gluteus medius and other gluteals in positions that simulate running. Activities that are done in this manner activate the entire functional kinetic chain of muscles and joints. The nonoperative sports medicine specialist, in particular the physiatrist and physical therapist, are in an excellent position to integrate treatment of the entire functional kinetic chain through a thorough biomechanical evaluation and comprehensive rehabilitation of the injured runner. Additional training in the areas of biomechanical evaluation and functional biomechanical deficits should be sought, because residency and even many fellowship-trained programs often overlook these important areas. Finally, the injured runner is best taken care of in a setting in which different sports medicine specialists are available and work well as a team. No one sports medicine specialist can provide all of the needs to the injured runner.

The Hip Flexors

Structure

The main muscles which draw the thigh-bone forward at the hip are known collectively as the hip flexor muscles. The two most important of these are iliacus and psoas major, which, although separate muscles, are given the combined name of iliopsoas, because their functioning is so closely interlinked.

Psoas major is attached to the front of the lumbar vertebrae, the lowest blocks of bone in your spinal column. It extends down across the front of your hip joint to fix onto a small bump of bone on the inside of the top of the thigh-bone, called he lesser trochanter. Iliacus spreads right over the inside of your hip-bone, round to the inner edge of the front of your sacrum. It extends down over the front of your hip joint, joining onto the outer side of psoas major tendon, so that it is fixed with the psoas tendon on he inner edge of the thigh-bone.

It is difficult to feel the hip flexors. The adductors form a fleshly covering over them at the top of the inner edge of the thigh-bone, and in the pelvis they lie under organs and the thick layers of your stomach muscles. In the groin, iliopsoas lies between the strong cords of sartorius and rectus femoris, which stand out over the front of the hip when you lift crease. But the hip flexors are crossed by a main artery ad nerve in the groin, so the discomfort you feel if you press your fingers over these structures prevents you from being able to feel the muscles moving when they contract to take your leg forward at the hip.

Functions

The hip flexors bend the thigh up at the hip, so they are working when you walk forward, and they have to contract harder when you run, especially up stairs or hilly ground. All forward kicking movements involve the hip flexors. If you lie on your back, and lift one leg up from the hip, with your knee bent or straight, the hip flexors perform the movement. If you lift both legs straight up in the air, lying on your back, you will feel your lower back tighten up into an arch, because psoas major fixes it attachment point on the vertebrae, in order to exert greater power in lifting the long lever of your legs. You will feel a similar effect in your lower back if you sit up with your back straight from lying flat. It is because of this tension effect i the back that double-leg-raising exercises in the forward direction can create back problems. In leg-raising exercises in the forward direction can create back problems. In leg-raising, the main work is done by the hip flexors, with the abdominal muscles stabilizing he trunk by contracting isometrically, so this type of exercise, which is often used to 'strength the stomach', is not even an effective way of doing that. Besides carrying the danger of damaging the back, it can cause a hernia in the abdomen or the groin.

The hip flexors also act to pull your lower back forward over your hips, for instance if you lie flat on your back and then sit up, keeping your back straight. When you sit upright on a chair or stool, your hip flexors work posturally to hold you, and counteract any tendency for your trunk to sway backwards. If your hip flexors are shortened or tight, whether as the result of injury or simply through your natural build, your lumbar spine will tend to curve more than the accepted normal, so that your back will be noticeably arched and hollow in its lowest part just above the pelvis. Problems with the hip flexors can relate directly to back problems, and can be either the cause or the result of spinal problems. This is especially true if the hip flexors on one side are shortened relative to the other side, for any reason. The asymmetry between the hips can cause distortion in the pelvis and lower spine, so that there is a functional imbalance. This can lead to over-strain during movements and activities involving the lower back.

Pain in the Groin

Problems in the hip-joint, or at the upper end of the thigh-bone, can cause grown pain. Back problems can cause referred pain over the front of the hip. These problems may involve mechanical strains inflammatory conditions, or disease processes. Your doctor has to distinguish between these various possible causes of your pain. Your accurate record of how the pain came on will help him to decide on which investigations would he appropriate, after he has examined you.

Inguinal Hernia

A fairly common cause of pain over the front of the hip is an inguinal hernia. The inguinal ligament is a band which crosses the top of your leg, almost exactly where the skin crease shows when you bend your leg at the hip. The ligament forms part of the containing tissue which divides your abdomen from your leg, and it is formed in parts, so that it contains 'gaps' through which nerves and other structures like the male spermatic cord can pass.

Too much pressure in your abdomen can force other tissues down through these gaps, so that they get caught on the wrong side of the separating ligaments: this is the hernia. The pressure in your abdomen is increased by such movements as lifting a heavy weight, especially if your bend forward as you lift, or lifting both legs straight up while you are lying on your back, or simply coughing or sneezing, so a hernia can be caused in a variety of situations. It can cause pain all the time, or only when your abdominal muscles contract to increase the pressure over the hernia. If the pain is intermittent, it may be difficult to distinguish from the pain of a muscle strain in the abdomen or hip flexors, so you have to keep a careful check of the pattern of the pain, and how it started, to help your doctor make the correct diagnosis.

If a diagnosed hernia causes a lot of pain, it is usually necessary to have an operation to replace the protruding tissue in its correct compartment in the abdomen, and to tighten up the gap through which it pushed. Progress back to sport after the operation is guided by the surgeon. Usually you start by straightening up gradually, as the pain makes you bend forward. As you begin to stand straighten, you start doing a gradually increasing amount of walking. At the same time, you start to try gentle and controlled stretching exercises for the abdominal and hip flexor muscles. As pain allows, you start jogging, then running, until you feel fit enough to resume sport.

You have to avoid heavy lifting, and any activities which might bring on a recurrence of the hernia. You can protect yourself by learning how to look after your back ad abdomen, for instance by bending your knees and keeping your back locked as straight as possible whenever you have to bend down to the floor, and especially if you have to lift even a light weight up.

Whenever you cough or sneeze, you should take care to keep your back stiff and straight. You should never do exercises which place a strong stomach, for instance isometric exercises like lying on your back and lifting both legs up straight. However, you should stretch your stomach and hip flexor muscles, to maintain good flexibility, ad you should actively strengthen these muscles with a dynamic exercises which do not create an excessive increase in abdominal pressure.

Self-help Measures for the Hip Flexors

(i) Rest it from any movements which cause pain. The probably means that you should avoid walking i the initial stages of the injury. It does not help you to use crutches, as you would have to hold your leg forward at the hip to do so, and you would therefore be working the injured hip muscles.

(ii) Once you have regained flexibility in the damaged muscles, you should start to use them, perhaps jogging, the gradually increasing speed, and finally by running up stairs and hills. If you play football, you can practice kicking a ball straight, against a wall, at a gradually increasing distance. You must take care to maintain full flexibility in the muscles while you begin to work them, and stretching should remain the first part of your warm-up and the last part of your warm-down whenever you do sport after you have recovered from the injury.

(iii) As quickly as possible after a traumatic strain, and as soon as an overuse strain has been diagnosed, you should start stretching the hip flexors. In the initial stages, this may involve no more than straightening your leg at the hip, while you are standing up, to counteract the tendency of the hurt muscles to shorten. As the pain decreases, you should gradually take your leg behind you, keeping your hip well forward, and holding the position at the point where you feel a 'pulling' sensation over the injury for a count of ten. As you regain flexibility in the muscles, you should then be able to place your injured leg behind you, and bend the forward knee increasingly, until you can hold the full-stretch position. At no stage should you push through the pain to increase the stretch over the muscles. Any increasing pain during or after stretching exercises means that you have forced the movement and over-stretched.

If the adductor muscles have also been injured, you must do stretching exercises for them too. Hip flexors stretching can also be combined with abdominal stretches, so the exercises are useful to add variety to your stretching programme.

(iv) Apply ice over the painful area, if the injury is sudden and severe.

(v) While you are unable to do your sport, you should use swimming as substitute exercise for fitness. Any stroke which does not cause pain is suitable, so you will probably find that, while you can swim crawl or breaststroke comfortably fairly soon after the injury happens, backstroke will be uncomfortable until the injury has almost healed.

A mild overuse strain may clear up within a couple of days, if you rest the injury from painful activities and start to stretch the muscles immediately. However, a severe strain may take between three and six weeks to be cured. During that period, you should feel progressively less discomfort, and more freedom of movement in the muscles, as you advance through the rehabilitation process. If your pain remains constant, or if you feel it at times when the muscles are completely at rest, you must suspect that there may be complications, so you should check back with your doctor for further investigations.

Injuries to the Hip Flexors Muscles

Extend of the damage

A sudden, very severe, shearing force can tear the hip flexors completely, where they form the tendon that attaches to the thigh-bone. Sometimes, the tendon may hold, but the lesser trochanter, the bump of bone to which the tendon is stuck, may be sheared away from the main thigh-bone. If the damage is severe enough to cause a total tear of the tendon, or an avulsion fracture in the bone, there is usually damage to the adductor tendon as well, and sometimes to other structures around the hip and the top of the thigh.

A less severe strain may cause a partial tear or over-stretch in the hip flexors. An overuse injury causes gradually increasing pain over the muscles, relating directly to the causative activity. On occasion, the injury may affect one of the bursae which lie under the tendons, rather than the tendons themselves.

What you feel

In a sudden severe strain, you feel a lot of pain over the hip flexors, which stops you from being able to draw your leg forward at the hip, and which creates discomfort when you take your leg back at the hip, stretching the hip flexors. Walking is difficult, but not impossible, and you may find that you lessen the discomfort if you turn your foot inwards or outwards as you walk. The degree of pain you feel is directly related to the amount of damage done, and the number of structures hurt, if other muscles and tissues besides the hip flexors are involved.

The gradually increasing pain of the overuse strain at first only comes on while you are doing the activity which has caused the injury. If you carry on with the activity, increasing the damage to the hip flexors, the pain increases, and you start to feel it whenever you work or stretch the muscles You may feel pain walking forward, and especially up stairs, or if you press your leg forward against a resistance, for instance by pressing your foot against a wall. The injured hip flexors will feel sore, and tighter than the other side, if you swing your leg backwards, or do exercises which stretch the front of the hip.

Causes

The hip flexors can be damaged by the same stresses which injure the adductors on the inner thigh. Your leg may be blocked as you take a kick in football or rugby. Your leg may be forced backwards at the hip by a tackle in football or hockey. If you catch your foot in a game like lacrosse, your trunk may be forced backwards over the hip.

Overuse strains happen to the hip flexors in long-distance running. The muscles perform most of the work of taking your leg forward at each step, so they can be strained simply by the fatigue of a distance run, or buy the extra effort of increasing your speed, or running up a hill. Any exercise directly involving the hip flexors can cause an overuse strain if you do too much of it. A sudden enthusiasm for double-leg-raising exercises lying on your back can strain the hip flexors or cause a hernia. Extended sessions of interval running up and down hills can strain the muscles. The same problem may arise if you suddenly start doing drills, such as kicking a football forward over and over again with the same leg, or practising run-ups for the pole vault.

Complications

An injury to the hip flexor muscles may coincide with any of the medical or inflammatory conditions that cause pain over the hip, so the diagnosis must be re-assessed if your pain does not resolve despite correct care. An avulsion fracture to the lesser trochanter may need surgery, if it causes continuing problems, and prevents functional healing. A more subtle complication may arise if the original injury causes you to adopt a bent-over posture at the hip. This can set up stress on the lower back, causing symptoms arising from the back as a secondary effect, which would not have been present at the time of the injury.

The Hip Joint

Structure

Functions

Your hip is a ball-and-socket joint. Your hip flexors bend your hip forwards; your glutei and hamstrings take your leg backwards; the hip abductors take it sideways; your adductor muscles take your thigh in towards and across your other leg; small muscles at the front of the joint turn your thigh-bone in towards your other leg, while similar muscles over the back of the hip twist your leg outwards.

Structurally, your hip is a very stable joint. It is tight enclosing capsule creates a negative pressure in the joint, which is further straightened by the ligaments and bone formation. Your hip helps to absorb shock takes through your legs or trunk, when you jump or fall down.

Functionally, your hips combine stability and motion. When you kick a ball, or balance in the ballerina's arabesque position, you pivot your whole weight over one hip, while the other hip creates free movement. Your hips co-ordinate with your pelvis and lower back, compensating for movement limitation due to the stability of the hips. If you do the splits, in either direction, your pelvis rotates, to achieve the movement, as your hips do not have enough freedom of movement to achieve such an extreme range.

Although your hips function as a pair, they are rarely symmetrical. You may be born with structural differences, or your postural habits may create these differences. If you lie on your back with your legs straight and completely relaxed, you may notice that one foot splays out sideways more than the other, indicating that rotation in one hip is greater than the other. You may notice that you can cross your legs more easily in one direction that the other when sitting. Or you may habitually stand with your weight resting over one hip when you are standing. When you do stretching exercises, you may find that some muscle grounds feel tight round one hip. If you notice this type of asymmetry, you must try to correct it by adopting good posture at all times, and stretching any tight muscles every day.

Bones

The rounded head of the top of the thigh-bone fits into a shallow cup-like formation called the acetabulum which forms part of the outer side of the hip-bone.

You cannot see or feel your hip joint, because it is covered with thick muscles. You can feel the prominent edge of the thigh-bone, called the greater trochanter, at the side of your hip. The trochanter forms the junction between the thigh-bone and its neck, which is directed inwards, and your hip joint is about six centimetres in towards your groin from the trochanter.

Soft tissues

Your hip is totally enclosed by a fibrous capsule, which is thickened over the front of the joint to form one of the strongest ligaments in the body, the iliofemoral ligament. Other ligaments protect the joint from behind ad underneath. A central ligament binds the middle of the thigh-bone head toi the acetabulum, but it is relatively weak, ad in some people it does not exist.

Hip Pain

Pain in the hip may be due to an inflammatory joint condition, which may affect only the one hip-joint, or it may be part of a syndrome affecting a number of joints with intermittent, unexplained pain. Osteoarthritis often affects the joint when you are older, because the hip is such an important weight-bearing joint, and therefore subject to hard wear-and-tear. Disease, such as tuberculosis, can affect the joint. Pain felt in the hip may be referred from other areas, such as the back, the groin, or the knee. A stress fracture at the upper end of the thigh-bone may also give a feeling of pain around the hip.

It is therefore very important to be able to describe to your doctor how your hip pain came on, when it occurs, and whether any particular movements make it worse or better. It my also be relevant to remember any other aches and pains in your legs and back. For adults, childhood problems in the hips or knees may have a bearing on later pain.

Hip Injuries

Because the hip-joint structure is so stable, it is rarely injured in itself through accidents i sports. You are much more likely to fracture your thigh or pelvis in severe injury than to disrupt the hip-joint. In children, however, structural defect in the hip-joint may become noticeable problems as the result of doing sport, although the problems are unlikely to have been caused by sport. In children and adults, the structures around the hip-joint may be injured during sports. In adults, the pain of osteo-arthritis may be felt most during sport, although it may also be evident at other times.

Bursitis

There are many bursae, or fluid-filled sacs for friction-free movement, around the hip-joint. They separate the tendons and other moving structures from the joint covering, so you find them at the front of the hip, under the hip flexor tendons, at the side, between the great trochanter and the iliotibial tract, and at the back, between the gluteal muscles and the joint. Where the bursa is close to the skin surface, as over the greater trochanter, it can be damaged by a direct low, if you fall over and hit the side of your hip, or if you are hit with a stick or bat. Otherwise, the most common cause of damage to the bursae is friction, usually from unaccustomed competitive movements, and sometimes due to muscle or tendon tightness, causing a loss of the free play in the tendon. Once the bursa is damaged, it becomes inflamed, and then sets up a very localized area of pain, which you feel when you press over the area, and when you move your leg in certain directions. It feels equally sore when the tendons over it are contracted or stretched, and thus helps to distinguish bursitis from a simple tendon strain. It also feels sore on direct pressure, so if you have bursitis under the gluteal muscles at the back of the joint, it hurts when you sit down on a hard chair.

To ease the discomfort, you can apply ice over the area, and gently stretch the tendons over the bursa. You must rest from any activities which cause or increase the pain. Your doctor may decide to treat the bursitis, possibly with an antiinflammatory injection. Once the soreness has gone, you can safely resume your sport, provided you do so gradually, and you try to avoid repeating the activity which caused the problem.

Perthes' Disease

This is a childhood problem affecting the hip-joint, and it usually happens to boys under the age of twelve. What happens is that the child's femoral head, in one or both hips, becomes flattened, and so no longer fits properly into the acetabulum on the hip-bone. This badly disrupts the working of the hip-joint, so the child starts to limp. What he feels, however, may be no more than a slight ache, which may happen either in the hip or in the knee. If the child is examined by a doctor, his hips will be visibly very limited i its movements, so the doctor will probably have X-rays taken which will reveal the extent ad nature of the problem. The cure is usually a period of total rest, until the bones in the hip-joint have recovered their normal shape. The sooner the diagnosis is made, the better and quicker the cure. If the problem is allowed to drag on for some time without being diagnosed, the long-term result is likely to be very early osteoarthritis in the joint, which may come on even as early as twenty to thirty years.

Osteoarthritis

Like all the joints we subject to loading, the hip is vulnerable to wear-and tear degeneration. Injuries to the hip in childhood make the joint more vulnerable to arthritis later on. A major injury like a slipped epiphysis which is not recognized and treated immediately can lead to arthritis before the age of thirty. More often, wear-and-tear arthritis comes on after the age of forty. In arthritis, the joint's cartilage surfaces are damaged, especially over the head of the femur. When the cartilage tries to heal itself, it forms a new rich blood supply, which in fact weakens the cartilage and the bone underneath it. This can lead to cysts forming in the bone, flattening of the head of the femur, and sometimes knobs of bone forming over the damaged area, which may break off into the joint, or which may stay stuck to the edges of the head of the femur.

When the degenerative process has developed to a severe stage it causes a gross limitation of movement, and usually a lot of pain. Your hip tends to be pulled inwards, and twisted, so that you can no longer take the joints through is full arc of movement. Pain in osteoarthritis can seem arbitrary. A lot of degeneration in the joint, which may sow up as gross changes on an X-ray, may cause no pain at all, while conversely minor degeneration may be very painful. If there is pain, heat will tend to make it worse, by increasing the blood flow into an already congested joint, so you will probably feel pain at night, if you sleep under very warm blankets. Most arthritis sufferers feel more pain in damp weather, because this causes changes in the pressure within the joint.

ORTHOPEDIC OVERVIEW

Traumatic injuries and overuse syndromes in the region of the pelvis, hip, and thigh are not as common as the frequently econountered knee, shoulder and elbow problems of the active athlete. A groin pull or a pelvic stress fracture, however, can be as devastating to an athlete as an anterior crusciate ligament tear.

Keep in mind as well that the anatomy in this region is complex. The patient's history, mechanism of injury, and symptoms may not provide sufficient information with which to formulate a diagnosis. Injured structures may be deep and difficult to palpate. Anatomic variations and overlying shadows frequently make interpretation of plain radiographs difficult, especially in the area of the pelvis, sacrum, and coccyx. It is for these reasons that orthopedic surgeons often find that additional imaging techniques are not only helpful but frequently crucial in order to pinpoint the exact diagnosis prior in initiating treatment.

Acute traumatic fractures and stress fractures of the pelvis and hip may be undetectable on routine radiographs. An adolescent with hip pain and a suspected early slipped capital amoral epiphysis may have normal radiographs. A young woman aerobic dancer with pubic symphysis pain and tenderness may have normal films as well. In both these cases, a triple phase bone scan in invaluable in helping to confirm or rule out the suspected diagnosis.

Injuries to the muscles and muscle attachments about the pelvis and hip are frequently quite difficult to isolate. The injured muscle may be small, deep, and well covered by more superficial layers of muscle and fat, making the physical exam less than diagnostic.

A skeletally immature gymnast may present with the sudden onset of anterolateral pelvic pain. The suspected diagnosis of an apophyseal avulsion injury may not be confirmed on plain films. A college long jumper experiences sudden thigh pain which prevents continued participation. A rectus femoris muscle disruption is suspected, but pain and swelling make the examination inconclusive. Imaging techniques which are currently available will be helpful in each of these cases. TPBS can provide information regarding increased blood flow or bone injury. CT scanning may clarify confusing radiographic findings in the situation of a bony avulsion injury. Magnetic resonance imaging may provide additional information regarding the extent and severity of muscle or tendinous disruption.

There are multiple bursas and tendons about the pelvis and hip which are subject to overuse. Trochanteric bursitis in a marathon runner or piriformis tendinitis in a ballet dancer can significantly impair function and performance. If these conditions do not respond promptly to the appropriate rest, anti-inflammatory medication, physical therapy, and perhaps steroid injection, then imaging in the form of bone scanning may be necessary to further localize and quantitate the inflammatory process.

An important issue regarding these imaging techniques centres on their clinical applicability. When and how are these diagnostic tests important to the treating physician? Certainly, not every pulled muscle warrants a bone scan or MRI. Some stress fractures can be clinically and radiographically proven without a bone scan. It is imperative, however, that we not allow an athlete to return to his or her activity in the face of a potentially serious problem. Often our active athletes become quite impatient with sports medicine physicians unless we are able to quickly make a diagnosis and institute effective therapy, allowing them to continue or resume their exercises promptly. At times, it is simply not possible to arrive at a diagnosis based on clinical evidence. It is at these times that modern imaging techniques offer invaluable assistance in the care of our patients.

Working closely with our radiologic colleagues is crucial. The radiologist must know the clinical question being asked by the treating physician in order to be able to recommend the most appropriate imaging modality.

Numerous surveys attest to the spectrum of traumatic and overuse injuries in this region of the body including specific entities that are age-related for adolescents, adults, and older athletes. The three separate anatomic areas of pelvis, hip, and thigh are combined as a unit in sport medicine primarily because of the large muscle groups that originate in the pelvis and serve the hip and thigh.

Modern imaging plays an important role in the diagnosis of abnormaltities in this region. Initial examination starts with the plain radiograph, which provides detailed images of the fine bony structure, which is crucial in the assessment of osseous injuries. Because of overlying structures in this region, computed tomography and magnetic resonance imaging allow the anatomic separation of otherwise confusing shadows. Triple-phase bone scanning is especially useful in patients with either acute injury or persistent chronic pain and with equivocal or normal radiographs. This is best demonstrated in the hip, where failure to diagnose an occult fracture can have serious and career threatening implications. Finally, TPBS offers the additional advantage of scanning large regions in a rapid fashion, allowing detection of unsuspected areas of pathology. One recent study utilizing TPBS for acute hip fractures found additional significant bony pathology, other than in the hip, in 41 per cent of patients.

The increased utilization of MR coupled with standard CT as well as three-dimensional CT has made these modalities valuable in the evaluation of sports medicine injuries in this region. Additionally, CT, when combined with standard imaging techniques, fluoroscopy, or arthorography, is particularly valuable for several specific diagnostic problems. CT and fluoroscopy are each useful in helping to localize intraarticular loose bodies and periarticular calcification. Arthrography combined with CT has been successful in helping to assess and localize ostecohondral fractures, to demonstrate capsule tear caused by earlier hip dislocation, and to aid in the diagnosis of illiopsoas baursitis.

Understanding the normal appearance of the hip demonstrated on CT and MR is essential to avoid misdiagnosing the normal as disease and in recognizing early disease entities. The recognition that the femoral head articulates with anterior, superior, and posterior articular surfaces of the acetabulum, forming a smooth, congruent articulating interface, is important. One most appreciate that the central area of the acetabulum contains fat and ligamentous structures which do not articulate with the femoral head in the same way that the peripheral bony articular rim does, in order to avoid possibly overcalling a centrally depressed acetabular fracture.

The MR appearance of the marrow about the hip undergoes evolutionary changes from early childhood through middle age and late adulthood. The capital femoral epiphysis contains fatty marrow as early as age 2 and demonstrates a bright signal intensity on T1-weighted images throughout life. This is in contrast to the proximal femoral metaphysis, which contains hematogenous marrow until late middle age and as such shows intermediate signal intensity on T1-weighted images until that time. Several normal areas of low-signal intensity are present, which include the bony residue of the former growth plate, the bridging trabecula within the proximal femoral metaphysis, the foveacentralis, and other anatomic features such as herniation pits of the femoral neck.

ACUTE PROBLEMS

Bony fracture/dislocation

Intertrochanteric hip fracture

Numerous studies have demonstrated the usefulness of TPBS in confirming suspected occult, acute fractures. Despite positive physical findings, these fractures may be radiographically unapparent, especially in difficult areas such as the hip, and, there fore, TPBS is especially helpful for these patients. Early detection of hip fracture has important economic, legal, and medical implications. This is particularly true for the athlete, since failure to correctly diagnose an occult hip fracture can be catstrophic and end a career. Intertrochanteric hip fractures have been found to have a characteristic appearance with TPBS. In patients with normal or equivocal radiographs, the sensitivity of TPBS was 97.8 per cent with a negative predictive value of 99 per cent. Of special interest was that other diagnoses including fractures of the pelvis, sacrum, tibia, spine, and rib were scintigraphically established in 41 per cent of patients. Additionally, meticulous imaging techniques and careful scan analysis enable us to differentiate less serious, focal fractures of the greater trochanter from intertrochanteric fractures.

Acetabular Fracture

Although plain film radiographs are mandatory in the assessment of possible acetabular fracture, difficulty in identifying and characterizing fractures, because of overlapping bony margins, has resulted in up to one-third of nondisplaced fractures being missed on the initial plain film examination. Detailed thin-section CT images through the acetabulum provide the maximum bony information available and do so without a necessity to move the patient. CT has virtually replaced conventional tomography for this purpose and should be performed on all patients with acetabular fracture.

Hip Dislocation

CT should be considered in the postoperative reconstructed pelvis to assure removal of intraarticular loose bodies as well as restoration of articular congruence. Occasionally, a patient may present with an irreducible dislocation of the hip. This may indicate that the femoral head has buttonholed through the capsule or that the pyriformis muscle has been displaced across the acetabulum, preventing relocation. Alternatively, an intraarticular loose body may be present, preventing relocation of a dislocated hip. Each of these entities may be diagnosed with CT. A major limitation of CT is its inability to visualize noncalcified carilage. In this setting, MR or a combined CT arthrogram may be diagnostic. Although there is always concern about exposing a young patient to ionizing radiation, a well-designed CT exam may frequently provide crucial diagnostic information at an integral radiation dose not than the plain film examination.

Typically, three types of hip dislocation are recognized: one directed posteriorly and two varieties anteriorly. The most common is the posterior dislocation of the femoral head, which is caused by impaction of the knee or tibia into a fixed object. From 8 to 15 percent of hip dislocations are in the anterior direction and include the iliopubic type as well as the less common obturator type. The diagnosis of these dislocations is usually apparent from the plain film examination. In difficult circumstances, however, the CT scan is diagnostic. Previous dislocation is also frequently accompanied by avulsion of the ligamenturm teres, which can be diagnosed with CT. Recurrent hip dislocation is quite infrequent, occurring in 0.3 to 1.2 per cent of cases.

Dislocations may be combined with tears of the joint capsule and of the cartilaginous labrum. Anterior dislocations are associated with anterior capsule tears and posterior dislocations with posterior capsule and/ or labrum tears. These entities can best be recognized with a combined CT arthrogram examination. Contrast injected into the joint space extravasates through the capsule or labral tear into the adjacent soft tissues.

This is usually easily seen on the associated CT exam.

Fractures of the Pelvis

Occult fractures of the pelvis are notoriously difficult to evaluate or confirm on plain film radiographs even when utilizing multiple oblique and lateral views. Fractures of the sacrumor cocyx as well as fracture/diastasis of the sacroiliac joint can be identified on TPBS and visualized in detail on CT exam.

MUSCLE INJURIES

Avulsion injuries

An apophysis is a secondary ossification center that contributes to the peripheral growth or contour of a bone but not to its longitudinal bone growth. Apophyseal avulsion injuries of the pelvis and hip in athletes are well documented in the literature. Adolescents are particularly susceptible to apophyseal avulsion injuries for two reasons. First, the pelvis and hip apophyses appear and fuse later than elsewhere in the body and are, therefore, open and susceptible during adolescence, generally 13 to 17 years old. Second, apophyseal avulsion is more likely than a muscle tear in adolescents, since it is the weakest point in the "mnusculotendinous unit".

The mechanism of injury is due to sudden muscle tension across an open apophysis. This occurs in one of two ways. Tension can be generated by sudden forceful concentric or eccentric contraction of a large muscle attempting to decelerate or accelerate the body. While this is the most common way for appophyseal avulsion, it can also occur after excessive passive lengthening of a muscle, as would occur in a cheerleader performing an anteroposterior split.

The displacement of the avulsed fragment is determined by the soft tissue attachments, which can prevent fragment migration as well as preserve muscle function by maintaining length. As the displacement of the fragment increases, there is more pain and muscle spasm. Avulsion fractures of the iliac crest and the anterior-inferior-iliac spine are, in general, less displaced, whereas avulsions of the ischium, anterior-superior iliac spine, and lesser trochanter show more fragment displacement. Treatment depends on the location of the avulsion as well as the degree of separation or attachment, and in some cases open reduction and internal fixation are necessary. Depending on the degree of displacement and/or healing, there can be a 3- to 5-cm shortening of the musculotendinous unit.

Clinically, these injuries usually occur as the result of an "extreme effort," and the athlete will usually complain of a popping, snapping, or tearing sensation as the avulsion occur. There is usually point tenderness and deep pain on palpation over the avulsion site. Radiographically, the injury is similar to a Salter-Harris I/II epiphyseal fracture. Each anatomic site has associated with it its own specific clinical features.

Muscle tear/bemorrhage

Muscle soreness accompanying or following extreme exertionis a common clinical symptom. Magnetic resonance imaging is useful in that setting, as T2-weighted sequences often show transiently increased signal within the affected muscles thought to represent muscle strain. When these findings are associated with an abnormal signal more than 3 weeks after injury or with perifascial hemorrhage, then muscle tear is the likely diagnosis. MR is especially useful in the diagnosis and follow-up of acute muscle hematoma, since no other imaging modality is as well suited to demonstrate the size of the hematoma or to follow its resolution.

Exertional Rbabdomyolysis

Rhabdomyolysis is a rare but sometimes catastrophic complication of severe exertional muscular trauma. Skeletal muscle injury due to exercise has been documented. There is disintegration or dissoclution of muscle associated with release of muscle fibre contents into the tissue fluid space and then eventually the circulation. A complication is the resulting myoglobiuria, which can lead to acute tubular necrosis and renal failure.

The damaged muscle can be identified on TPBS with the mechanism of uptake similar to that seen with myocardial infarct scanning, whereby there is an influx of calcium ions into acutely necrotic muscle cells, which then bind with the phosphate from the technetium scanning agent. The bone scanning agent shows increased uptake in areas of pain that is best visualized at 48 h after injury and virtually undetectable at 1 week. In addition to the clinical and TPBS findings, there are also laboratory values which in clude increase in serum CK levels.

CHRONIC PROBLEMS

Overuse injuries (stress fractures/periostitis)

Stress fractures of the hip and pelvis are similar to those in other parts of the body. A continuum exists beginning with early bone remodeling continuing through subclinical stress fracture and terminating in clinical stress fracture. TPBS has been shown to be exceptionally sensitive in detecting and localizing areas of overuse injury. This is especially important, since studies have shown that positive radiographic findings in femoral neck stress fractures may lag behind symptoms for as long as 2 to 4 weeks. The team physician must have a high clinical index of suspicion and should pursue additional imaging tests even if plain radiographs remain normal.

Hip and Femur

In McBryde's study of 1000 consecutive fractures in runners, 14 per cent were found in the femur. Undetected femoral neck fractures have a potential for displacement with resulting serious complications such as nonunion, malunion, and in some cases eventual aseptic necrosis. Although quite uncommon, bilateral femoral stress fractures have also been reported. Many biomechanical studies have been performed demonstrating and measuring the large loads transmitted through the femur. Experimental studies have shown that just walking exerts forces through the femur equivalent to six times body weight, while running and jogging can increase these peak forces to 10 to 20 times body weight. The highest area of strain was noted to be in the calcar area of the femur. Additional studies have been able to identify two doscrete types of femoral neck stress fractures with specific clinical features identified with each one.

As with stress fractures in other regions of the body, MR demonstrates characteristic findings. There is diminished signal in the affected portion of the bone on T1-weighted images and high signal in those same areas on T2-weighted images. These findings represent edema and/or hemorrhage into the involved bone and indicate underlying stress fracture. With long-standing overuse, such as in marathon runners, there may be accentuation of the trabecular pattern causing diminished signal intensity in the involved area on both T1- and T2-weighted images. When a completed fracture occurs, the magnetic resonance scan shows a linear area of diminished signal on T1-weighted images in the area corresponding to the fracture line.

Despite loss of vascularity and impending avascular necrosis, the femoral head continues to look normal for at least 48 h and likely for at least 5 days following interruption of blood supply. The predominant marrow present in the femorla head is fatty in composition. From 2 to 5 days is required for necrotic changes to occur within fatty marrow.

TPBS is the most common imaging modality to identify femoral neck stress fractures. In athletes, compression-type fracture involving the concave portion of the neck is the most common type, explaining the bone scan finding of focal, intense, rounded area of activity limited to this portion of the femoral neck. High-resolution delayed images are the most helpful, and very often only routine anteroposterior views are needed. However, if the suspected stress fracture is not identified on this view, then additional views, such as the frog-leg view, magnification view, computer-assisted subtraction view, or SPECT imaging, must be utilized. Additionally, serial scans can be used to follow up femoral neck stress fractures.

In summary, pubic stress fractures are mechanical disruptions of the bones of the pelvis from excessive, repetitive muscular activity or stress at the ischiopubic ramus, which is the origin of external hip rotators and adductors of the hip joint. Similarly, this type of injury has also been reported in soldiers.

In a study by Noakes et al., there is a clinical triad seen in marathon or long-distance runners with pelvic stress fractures: (1) severe groin pain preventing any running activity, (2) positive standing sign, (3) severe, exquisite pain on deep palpation of the inferior pubic ramus. Radiographs are only infrequently positive in pelvic stress fracture, whereas the TPBS is invariablydiagnostic. When the radiographs are positive, they will reveal a nondisplaced fracture of the inferior pubic ramus. TPBS reveal a single or focal "hot spot" in the same area, which so characteristic for a stress fracture. This is in contrast to traumatic or overuse osteitis pubis, which shows diffuse nonspecific bilteral uptake. This very specific and unique pelvic/ pubic stress fracture commonly seen in female long-distance and marathon runners occurs at the origin of the gracilis muscle and has been termed the gracilis syndrome.

Another pelvic overuse problem is the pyriformis syndrome, involving spasm and pain along the course of this muscle which has the scieatic nerve running along its lower border and occasionally with the muscle itself. This muscle, which is an external hip potator and thigh abductor, has its origin from the anterior surface of the sacrum, the anterior capsule of the sacroiliac joint, and the gluteal surface of the ilium. It exits the pelvis through the greater sciatic foramen and inserts on the superior border of the greater trochanter. This syndrome is thought to result from overuse, with a history of trauma identified in only 50 per cent of the cases. Patients present with buttock or low back pain and normal radiographs. The none scan shows a linear band of increased activity along the entire course of the muscle.

Thigh

In the midthigh, there is an unusual and unique overuse syndrome associated with periostitis at the insertion of the adductor muscles. Thigh splints, or adductor insertion avulsion syndrome, is to the thigh what shin splints is to the tibia. Primarily reported in female military recruits, it appears to be associated with continued forced overstriding and the resulting periostitis and characteristic TPBS appearance.

Bursitis

Burstitis is often a diagnosis made by exclusion. Radiographs are normal, and TPBS, CT, or MR imaging is performed to identify the chronic cause for hip or groin pain in order to exclude a more serious entity such as a stress fracture.

Trochanteric bursitis has a very subtle but typical TPBS pattern of increased curvilinear uptake either at or adjacent to the greater trochanter on blood pool and delayed images. This entity can be seen in athletes of all ages and shows a pattern which is clearly distinct from femoral neck stress fracture, intertrochanteric fracture, greater trochanger fracture, or degenerative arthritis of the hip.

The iliopsoas bursa is a normally occurring structure which, when enlarged, may present as a painful groin mass. Enlargement is often associated with preexisting joint abnormality. Diagnosis may be suspected on CT or MR examination and confirmed with a combined CT arthrogram. The iliopsoas bursa lies posterior to the iliopsoas tendon and lateral to the femoral vessels and overlies the hip joint capsule between the pubocapsular and iliocapsular ligaments. Communication of the iliopsoas bursa with the hip joint occurs in 9 to 15 per cent of patients.

Avascular Necrosis

CT, MR, and nuclear bone scans have each been used to provide important diagnostic information concerning avascular necrosis. A number of studies report a high level of diagnostic accuracy provided by these modalities. Recent reports suggest that MR is the most sensitive and accurate modality in the early diagnosis of avascular necrosis of the femoral head with an accuracy in the range of 94 per cent. Since prognosis may be related to early treatment, the diagnosis of avascular necrosis before radiographic findings occur may be beneficial. Ficat devised a commonly used staging system for avascular necrosis. In the earliest stage 0 disease, patients are asymptomatic with normal radiographs and normal nuclear bone scans but with a positive MR scan. At that stage, there is some evidence to suggest that early treatment may prevent progression of the disease.

Typically, avascular necrosis presents with a variety of magnetic resonance imaging patterns. Commonly, a linear area of diminished density of a ring a of diminished density at T1-weighted sequences is seen. With T2-weighting, an inner border of high-signal intensity may be seen in up to 80 per cent of cases. Edema within the bone marrow may b an early feature. This is nonspecific and may also be seen with transient osteoporosis, early stress fracture, occult fracture, and osteomyelitis. Joint effusion causing distention of the joint capsule is a nearly constant finding.

In advanced cases of avascular necrosis, magnetic resonance and computed tomography both show femoral head flattening with subcortical compression fracture. Numerous studies have compared the relative accuracy of nuclear bone scanning, MR, and bone marrow pressure measurement in the diagnosis of avascular necrosis of the femoral head.

DIAGNOSTIC PROBLEMS

Infection

Septic arthritis and osteomyelitis are urgent medical/surgical problems that can often mimic athletic injuries. A combination of TPBS, CT, and/or MRI can be utilized to secure the diagnosis.

Vascular

Arterial and venous problems of the pelvis and

thigh associated with pain and swelling can present diagnostic difficulty in athletes. Until the last 5 years, contrast venography was the imaging tool of choice in diagnosing thrombophlebitis, but Doppler sonography has now replaced this as the test of choice, and in some circumstances CT can also identify the defect. The blood flow phase of TPBS is primarily intended to identify athletic injuries that are acute and relatively hyperemic in nature. Occasionally and incidentally, arterial/venous abnormalities and malformations are noted and then pursued in greater detail by MRI or angiography.

Bone Tumor

Benign or malignant bone lesions can mimic athletic injuries and have been, therefore, termed as sports tumours in the literature.

Slipped femoral Capital epiphysis

This entity occurs in the 9 to 17-year-old age group, with the problem representing a shift of movement of the femoral head on the shaft. Although the exact cause is not known, it is thought to be nontraumatic in nature. The resulting pain, often referred to the thigh or knee, is the most frequent clinical complaint and often associated with a limp. On radiographs, there is widening of the radiolucent growth plate on the affected side, and the epiphysis of the involved femoral head is slightly displaced dorsally and/or medially. The TPBS pattern is quite specific, reflecting the response to abnormal movement of the growth plate of the affected side appearing as increased activity in this are on both blood pool an high-resolution delayed images.

13

THE IMPORTANCE OF TAPING AND BRACING IN SPORTS INJURIES

INTRODUCTION

A frequent question asked by the injured athlete to the sports medicine practitioner is "How should I protect this injury once I return to play?" The answer should result from a decision-making process, dependent on several factors. One of these factors is the knowledge and awareness of what is available. It is the sports medicine practitioner is exposed to numerous taping techniques and braces that may be beneficial in meeting the needs of athletic patients. If is not the authors' intent to teach competence in the techniques of taping or the designing of a brace, however, some detailed examples are presented to aid the discussion. The ability of the physician to identify and evaluate the options will facilitate prescription of the optimal method of support and protection. This understanding will also assist in communication to coaches, trainers, and therapists working with the athlete, thus encouraging the team approach, a necessary component of optimal patient care.

SELECTION CONSIDERATIONS

Before considering common methods of athletic injury support, it is helpful to discuss factors to consider in making an appropriate selection, including: (1) diagnosis of injury, (2) goals to be accomplished by taping or bracing, (3) resources available, (4) sport and position of the athlete, (5) the athlete's acceptance, (6) research findings, and (7) personal preferences. The investigation of these factors and how they interact will assist in the tors and how they interact will assist in the process of determining the best solution.

Diagnosis of Injury

The location, nature, and severity of injury often dictate the suitability of providing external support. For instance, most shoulder problems are not helped by taping or bracing since restriction of range of motion leads to decreased function and possibly secondary problems. However, the ankle, with its inherent skeletal stability, may be more readily supported by external support. The acuteness and severity of injury may dictate more aggressive treatment than taping or bracing can achieve. Some chronic injuries may be helped by decreasing the effect of biomechanical forces on repetitive activities. A referral to and input from an orthopaedist may be beneficial.

Goals of Taping and Bracing

Taping and bracing can be divided into three main categories: (1) prophylactic, (2) rehabilitative, and (3) functional. Prophylactic supports are used to reduce the incidence or severity of injury to uninjured normal anatomy or fully rehabilitated injuries. Rehabilitative taping, or bracing is used to provide protection of healing injuries during their rehabilitation. Functional braces and taping are used to protect against reinjury following rehabilitation and/or surgical reconstruction. A taping procedure or brace effective for prevention may not be suitable as an adjunct to rehabilitation. Taping or bracing does not substitute for the need for complete rehabilitation. A helpful concept is that of "earning the brace" by completing the rehabilitation. Taping may act as an adjunct to help support injured tissues during rehabilitation; it is a means to an end, not the end itself. If taping or bracing cannot provide any additional benefit, it is probably best to do without it.

Resources Available

Even though a certain taping technique may be ideal for a particular problem, it will not help if there is no trainer or other individual skilled in its application available to the athlete. This is a key advantage to many braces. Once the athlete is properly instructed in their application, no additional expertise is needed. Also, there are financial considerations such as the cost of taping and the often times considerable investment required to purchase a brace. With custom-made braces, there may be a period of time before the brace is available for the athlete's use. Coaches and trainers should be approached to determine which options are feasible. In the case of younger athletes, parents should be involved when financial or insurance issues need clarification.

Sport and Position

A taping or bracing that is effective for an athlete in one sport may not be suitable for another athlete, or even the same athlete in another sport. Each sport has it own physical requirements, equipment, environment, and rules that will affect, and many times govern, the selection of protective support for injuries. In some sports, and athlete's particular position or event may need to be considered. Taping may have to be tailored to allow the athlete to perform his or her skills, yet provide adequate protection. Braces must be made of materials that do not endanger the other participants.

Athlete's Acceptance

If the athlete feels that taping or a brace is uncomfortable or decreases performance, the attempt to support an injury will fail. Involving the athlete in the decision-making process and providing choices, where possible, reduce the risk of nonacceptance. If an appropriate choice is made, a very real effect of taping or bracing following injury is the psychological assistance to the athlete's confidence upon returning to competition.

Research Findings

Research about what does and does not work is still in the infancy stage. Many methods and devices that have been used for years have never been tested rigorously. With respect to new techniques or products, it is probably best to keep an open mind but to be critical. Until more work is done, clinical experience will have to suffice.

Personal Preference

After gaining clinical experience with various taping techniques and braces, one usually begins to have certain favourites. There is nothing wrong with relying on experience when the athlete is looking for expert answers, as long as each case is viewed individually.

IMPLEMENTATION

TAPING

To be proficient in taping, one must practice. Anyone who has attempted to learn to tape knows how true this statement is. However, exposure to some common techniques can assist the primary care practitioner in providing a complete treatment plan and in being able to communicate with professionals skilled in these methods. After discussing basic principles, as sampling of common taping methods is presented.

Principles of Taping

Application

One of the most common mistakes made by the

novice is applying too much tape. Every piece of tape should have a distinct purpose—more is not better. Other common problems are continuous application of tape and forcing the tape to go in a desired direction; these errors may restrict circulation. A better approach consists of tearing strips often and considering the contours of body parts. Learning how to tear tape and adapting two-dimensional tape to a three-dimensional body part are basic skills. A good taper keeps in mind the need to restrict undesired motion yet allow wanted motion. A tape support is made effective by bridging across the injury and duplicating the anatomy needing support; strength is developed by weaving the strips, overlapping by at least one-half the width of the tape.

Tape Selection

Another important principle is the correct selection of the best tape for the job. The size of the body part determines the appropriate width. The tape must have good adherence to the athlete's skin and have adequate tensile strength to provide the necessary support. Some tapes have elasticity to allow increased ease of application or desired movement, yet provide adequate injury protection; of course this increases it cost. Of importance to the taper is how the tape unwinds from the roll and how easily it tears. Learning how to tear tape is the most basic skill learned by the novice taper. Some tapes do not tear and require cutting between application of strips.

Skin Care

Frequent taping of skin can lead to problems that are preventable. Shaving hair not only increases the effectiveness of taping but also reduces the irritation and buildup of residue that can lead to infection. Skin to be taped should be protected by application of a taping base that also increases the adherent qualities of the tape. A tape underwrap of thin polyester urethance foam decreases skin problems while it increases the athlete' comfort; however, this adds another interface between the tape and the structure needing support. A lubricant placed in areas that may be pinched with movement within the taping, such as the lace and hell areas of the ankle, can prevent of at least decrease irritation. Correct removal of the tape, using appropriate scissors or cutters, should be taught to the athlete. Scissors with pointed tips should be avoided. Following practice, the skin must be thoroughly cleansed and treated if necessary. Failure to do so can lead to skin breakdown and wounds that may prevent further taping. Some individuals may develop allergic reactions to certain products of materials used in taping, and solutions to this problem must be found. If not, taping may need to be abandoned in favour of some other form of support and protection.

Procedures

This section describes and presents some common uses of tape to support athletic injuries. It is not intended to be complete or exhaustive but rather to reflect current practice.

Buddy Taping

This method splints an injured finger to an adjacent finger to restrict varus/valgus forces. For additional support, felt or foam may be placed between the fingers being taped. It is important to allow interphalangeal motion and to avoid using the index and little fingers as a splint, unless, of course, either is the finger involved.

Thumb Figure-of-Eight

Hyperflexion injuries are supported by circling around the wrist and the thumb in a figure-of-eight pattern.

Thumb Checkrein

Hyperextension injuries to the thumb may be aided by the use of a checkrein between the thumb and index finger. Please note that use of this taping can result in injuries to the metacarpophalangeal joint of the index finger.

Wrist Taping

Circumferential strips about the wrist may limit excusion of the carpals. In cases of dorsal impingement such as in the gymnast or tennis player, the incorporation of a foam "block" into this taping is often helpful.

Elbow Hyperextension Taping

With the athlete's elbow placed in slight flexion, fanning strips are placed anterior to the elbow joint between anchors about the upper arm and forearm. This taping can be modified to also provide medial or lateral support.

Shoulder Taping

Although taping has been and can be used for some shoulder injuries, we feel that the restriction of motion required to provide adequate support decreases function to a point where time and effort are probably spent on rehabilitation.

Hip and Groin Taping

These areas are better supported by the use of elastic wraps using a figure-of-eight pattern about the waist and upper thigh. Since these areas are rarely taped, no further discussion is presented. Again, the question of decreased function to achieve the desired support is important.

Medial Knee Taping

Fanning strips across the medial aspect of the knee

joint across anchors about the thigh and calf may reduce the effect of valgus stress.

The next three taping procedures are presented in a step by step manner. They are not easily demonstrated by a single photograph. They address areas where external support is most often considered.

Knee Anterior Cruciate Ligament (ACL) Taping

The Duke Simpson knee strapping has often been touted: "If this strapping fails to hold a knee from further sprain, no brace or other contrivance will." Using a modification of this strapping, Ross developed an effective method to limit hyperextension of the knee, a major factor in anterior cruciate ligament injury. The modification shown here uses a four-tailed piece of neoprene rubber, 15" × 6" with 5" × 3" triangular cutouts. Tape adherent and underwrap are applied, the neoprene support placed in the popliteal space and then covered by underwrap. This is done to enable the athlete to reuse the neoprene. Using 3" elastic tape, a circumferential anchor is placed about the calf, revolving laterally.

The tape is drawn laterally and upward across the lateral joint line. A circumferential anchor about the thigh is then placed. Continuing on the medial side, the tape is drawn downward across the medial joint line, around the calf, then upward across the medial joint line again. The creates a medial "X" and covers the neoprene support. After passing the tape around the thigh, then down across the lateral joint line, the lateral "X" is completed. After passing behind the calf again, the tape is pulled laterally, then upward and posteriorly.

This should enclose the popliteal space, a practice not usually done due to circulatory problems encountered. The use of the neoprene support seems to counter this problem. After completing a finishing anchor about the thigh, the tape is cut and, cloth adhesive tape placed about the thigh and calf to anchor the elastic tape. These anchors and the edges of the elastic tape should be applied directly to the skin. Cutting the calf portion of the taping posteriorly allows for expansion of the gastrocnemius musculature. This gap is closed with cloth adhesive tape to finish the taping. In order to recover the neoprene support for reuse, this taping is removed strip by strip upon conclusion of activity.

Ankle Taping

Although there are probably about as many taping techniques for the ankle as there are trainers, a basic method that incorporates some of the most common methods will be described. To meet goal of the taping—preventive, rehabilitative, or supportive for a functional return of a rehabilitated ankle injury—the basic steps are adapted by the experienced taper. The athlete's ankles should be positioned at a right angle of plantar/ dorsiflexion with neutral inversion/eversion. Hair should be shaved to provide maximal support. Heel and lace pads made of gauze or similar protective material with lubrication are applied to the heel and lace areas to guard against blisters and tape cuts.

Tape adherent and underwrap are then applied. Under wrap may be omitted to provide additional support, especially for more acute injuries, but special care of the skin is then required. Anchor strips around the calf at the level of the musculotendineous junction of the gastroc-soleus and around the arch are applied.

The arch anchor must be placed proximal to the base of the fifth metatarsal to avoid discomfort as the foot spreads with weight bearing. A "stirrup" strip is placed on the calf anchor medially, passing beneath the heel posterior to the malleoli, pulling laterally to the other side of the calf anchor. In an eversion sprain, the stirrup is placed with equal tension medially and laterally. Perpendicular to the stirrup, a "horseshoe" is applied distal to the malleoli, starting and finishing on the arch anchor. Strirrups and horseshoes are repeated twice more, overlapping the previous strip by one-half. This completes the "basketweave". A "figure-of-eight" may be applied to restrict plantar flexion. In the present example, it begins on the outside of the foot, angling under the foot. "Heel locks" are used to restrict inversion/eversion. A medial heel lock, restricting inversion, begins in the lace area, angling behind and across the medial aspect of the heel, then under the heel and returning the lace area. A lateral heel lock is performed in the opposite direction, angling across the lateral aspect of the heel. These steps may be repeated as necessary to obtain the desired support.

Circularstrips are placed about the lower leg, overlapping distal to proximal, to eliminate open spaces that may result in skin irritation or blisters. Anchors may be repeated to close, thus decreasing the number of free tape ends exposed that may roll up when the athlete puts on socks. The complete job is inspected for wrinkles and gaps, and the athlete questioned as to the adequacy of the support and its comfort. The ankle strapping is removed by using a blunt-nosed bandage scissors or tape cutter to cut along the medial aspect, posterior to the medial malleous. Various padding may be incorporated into the taping, such as a "J" pad along the lateral malleolus for subluxation of the peroneal tendons, or a dorsal "block" in the lace area to restrict dorsiflexion in cases of anterior impingement.

Frequently, questions are asked about the value of

preventive ankle taping. A review of the literature by Metcalf and Denegar highlights several points. With exercise, the initial restriction of range of motion is considerably reduced, but does appear to be adequate to restrict the extreme ranges of motion responsible for ankle injury. There are some who feel that the restriction of ankle movement may increase the incidence of knee injuries, but this has been refuted by research. Ankle taping does affect athletic performance. There is some evidence that the protective effect of taping is due to increased proprioceptive input. It appears that the use of ankle taping to prevent reinjury to ankles previously injured is more easily defended. Also there is some benefit, albeit less, from the use of reusable cloth ankle wrapping or a high top shoe. The greatest issue is that of cost benefit. Until it can be conclusively established that the cost of labour and supplies needed to provide protective taping outweighs the cost of preventable injury, the decision of whether or not to tape will rely on professional opinion and budget considerations.

Arch

This taping method may be effective to control to control excessive pronation, to decrease stress on the plantar fascia, and as an adjunctie treatment for shin splint. Due to the increased perspiration of the soles of the feet, it is almost mandatory to apply this taping without the use of underwrap. An anchor strip is placed loosely around the metatarsal heads. These steps are repeated once or twice. Next horizontal strips are placed, pulling medially, from the heel to the ball of the foot. A "low dye" strip is begun at the base of the little toe, passed behind the heel, and then ended at the base of the great toe. A closing anchor is placed on the dorsum of the foot over the original anchor. Care must be taken to account for the expansion of the foot upon weight bearing.

Achilles Tendon Taping

This taping uses anchors around the arch of the foot and the calf with elastic tape to give support to the musculotendinous structure. The athlete's ankle is taped in a position of slight plantar flexion, thus restricting excessive dorsiflexion.

Furf-Toe Taping

Strips are fanned between anchors around the great toe and the arch to prevent flexion and/or extension of the great toe.

BRACING

The primary care practitioner can become overwhelmed when attempting to choose a brace. The bracing market is full of claims with no guarantees, just disclaimers of liability. Often the athlete may already have a brace or knows of someone from whom to borrow one. The physician's role is then to evaluate critically the brace's effectiveness. With new products available every day, it is probably more important to recognize certain features of the common braces. After presenting some of the advantages and disadvantages of bracing, a discussion of some presently available functional braces and orthotics follows.

Bracing—Pros and Cons

When compared with taping, there are several advantages to bracing. First and foremost is ability to provide protection or support to athletes who do not have access to a skilled taper. Also once the initial investment is made, braces may be more cost effective. In certain problems, a brace or orthotic device can provide a means of support not available from taping. Most braces are more convenient, but drawbacks do exist. Because of the additional interface and lack of adhesion to the skin, the problem of migration can occur during vigorous activity. This may led to failure of the brace to provide support and also cause decreased athletic performance or other problems. The use of tape adherent, anti-migration straps, or specially designed undergarments may help. The most common complaint made by the athlete is the weight some braces require to provide adequate protection. With wear, Velcro fasteners fail to hold fast, straps or buckles break, and elastic stretches out. Waiting for replacement parts does not allow the athlete to participate safely without the brace. Another problem is sizing—what do you do with athletes who are between sizes or have body proportions differing from the brace design? Custom-made braces are available but are generally more expensive. The best advice is to select devices carefully and to be prepared to deal with the problems that may arise from the brace prescribed to protect the patient. This is an area where you may need to seek the advice of the trainer, sports therapist, or orthotist.

SUGGESTIONS FROM OUR PRACTICE

Tennis Elbow Strap

Epicondylitis is most commonly seen in athletes in racquet sports, baseball, and softball who perform repeated forearm pronation and supination movements. The sports medicine practitioner can supplement and augment the rehabilitation program with a Velcro or elastic strap combination brace often called a "tennis elbow strap" or "counter-force brace." There are numerous braces of this type on the market designed to reduce the contractile force of the extensor musculature, which causes irritation and inflammation at or near the radiohumeral joint.

Silicone Rubber Wrist/Hand Cast

Some hand and wrist injuries requiring immobilization may be supported so that participation in sports is permitted, even in collision sports such as football. By fabricating a playing cast out of various silicone rubber compounds, the injury can be given adequate protection without subjecting other participants to risk from an unyielding material. Details of their construction are found in the references.

Lateral Prophylactic Knee Braces

Prophylactic lateral knee braces, designed to lessen the severity of lateral impact, valgus force injuries, are still in relative in fancy both in design and implementation. Recent research has raised questions as to the possibility of "preloading" knee structures and predisposing the wearer to an increased risk of ligament injuries. Brace migration is a major problem as is compliance of the athlete in proper positioning and care of the brace, all essential to the successful success of effectiveness by: (1) shaving the skin as described for taping, (2) using a taping adherent, (3) using audiovisual aids supplied by the manufacturers in teaching proper application and for daily reminders, (4) daily checking of positioning by coaches and trainers, and (5) weekly checking on upkeep by coaches, parents, equipment managers, trainer, and players.

As with all braces, with lateral prophylactic knee braces there is no guarantee that an injury will not occur, but rather an assumption that, by design, lateral impact injuries may be lessened in severity. A practical problem faced by the sports medicine practitioner is the popularity of the braces based on anecdotal reports of bent braces that "saved" a player from injury, but research has not substantiated this claim. Hewson et al., found that in collegiate football players there appeared to be no reduction in the number of knee injuries since the adoption of lateral prophylactic knee braces and subsequent rule changes. With respect to their effect on performance, Prentice and Toriscelli found that there was a significant decrease in 40yard-dash times while wearing the braces but no decrease in agility or backward running.

We feel that time and money might be better spent on preventive conditioning than on braces for now, in light of recent research. Lateral knee braces may have a place at the end of a total rehabilitation program, but the popular axiom that the lateral knee braces are "better than nothing," in view of recent research to the contrary for athletes without injury, may require rethinking.

Functional Knee Braces

Another recent surge in brace development is that of functional knee braces. These are designed to provide support knees made unstable by in jury or to provide additional protection following surgery to correct these instabilities. Some of these braces are "read-made," with sizing to provide for immediate fit. Others require custom construction based on some form of cast molding or measurement of the athlete's leg. Considering the condition being addressed and the cost of these devices, input from the orthopedist is critical. Attempts to support anterior cruciate injuries usually involve some form hyperextension stop through the use of controlled hinges and control of the rotational component through the use of straps or fitted shells. These braces also provide support to other knee structures. Some studies have investigated the relative effectiveness of these braces, but no brace has been found to completely control the knee in all situations.

Knee Bracess for Patellofemoral Pain Syndromes

Peripatellar pain and/or dysfunction resulting from anatomical causes, otherwise known as extensor mechanism malalignment is being more accurately diagnosed and treated as knowledge of patellofemoral mechanics is increased by research. We have found success with two types of braces in assisting the athlete in return to full function, the Palumbo lateral patella stabilizing brace, and the neoprene rubber sleeve with patellar cutout.

The Palumbo brace combines the support of an elastic sleeve with patellar cutout with a lateral buttress strap designed to dynamically decrease excessive lateral tracking of the patella, which is commonly responsible for the pain experienced by patients with EMM. Lysholm et al., reported that during isokinetic testing of patients with EMM in braced and unbraced conditions, strength measurements increased while pain decreased during the test with the patellofemoral joint braced.

Neoprene braces provide uniform compression and allow for nearly normal range of motion of the knee. It is essential that the athlete with EMM or patellar tendinitis be fitted with a sleeve with a cutout for the patella. This is necessary to allow full range of motion, support, proper tracking, and decrease compression of the patellofemoral joint with activity. There are numerous brands available, some with a lateral buttress, for the physician and athlete to choose from, always keeping in mind the need for a patellar cutout.

Knee Sleeves

Sleeves can be used to provide compression of the knee as well as other soft tissue areas, such as the calf musculature and the quadriceps and hamstrings. They are often made of elastic or Spandex and provide even compression and may promote local tissue healing. Neoprene is another material used for these purposes. It major difference from elastic and Spandex is its ability to retain body heat, thereby increasing the sense of warmth that sometimes makes the athlete who suffers from tendinitis more comfortable. They also provide some pain relief from sensory stimulation. Patients wearing these devices report a feeling of security, probably due to increased proprioceptive input. As discussed previously, when a sleeve is used at the knee it is important to use a brace that has a patellar cutout to decrease irritation to those prone to EMM.

Ankle Braces

Numerous ankle braces are available commercially which provide the sports medicine practitioner variety and flexibility in fitting the individual athlete and to support the injury. Slip-on elastic braces are best utilized when even compression is desired, such as to decrease oedema. They do not restrict inversion or eversion significantly enough to be considered prophylactic support. Certain manufacturers combine the comfort of even compression using Spandex, elastic, and Velcor strap combinations to restrict inversion or eversion. We have found them easier to manage with regard to the break-in period and they are a better alternative than the slip-on ankle brace. A third type of prophylactic support for the ankle is a lace-up style. These braces often have medial and lateral stays, providing increased restriction of inversion or eversion motions. In considering the use of these braces, one might also consider them as an alternative or adjunct to ankle taping, especially if a competent, skilled taper is not readily available. Bunch et al., compared the comfort and effectiveness of ankle taping to five different commercial ankle braces. Initial comfort and support were highest in the freshly taped ankle. However, after 20 minutes of inversion exercises, "two of the lace on braces offered the same level of support as the tape." They concluded that, at the end of their conservative 20-minute test, there was no difference in the level of support for the top two lace-on style braces and taping.

Air Cast

The air cast can be of great use to the physician, therapist, and trainer from early in the rehabilitation program to the late stages of return to functional activity for the athlete with a moderate to severe ankle injury. Stover described the use of a semirigid support in case studies of seven athletic patients. The air cast is similar in design and principles for use to the semi-rigid material described. It provides a milking effect upon weight bearing, which appears to decrease post-trauma edema with the addition of an air bag lining, it allows for an earlier return to functional activities, it decreases unwanted excessive inversion and eversion, and it protects the already injured lignamentous and soft tissues from reinjury or further injury, thereby decreasing rehabilitation time. We have found that air casts are easy to use and fit in most athletic footwear. Their application is easily taught and followed and the athlete's confidence in the brace is increased with use. Even when combined with ankle taping, it does not significantly decrease speed or jumping ability.

SHOE INSERTS

Although not truly braces, orthotics are common devices used to aid in the treatment of athletic injury. Orthotics are defined here as devices placed in the athlete's shoe to balance the foot during activity. External support in the area of orthotics requires careful selection by the practitioner and athlete alike, always being conscious of the demands of the activity, ease of application, and adaptability to the athlete's condition.

Soft Orthotics

Sometimes used until the permanent orthotic returns from the laboratory, some soft orthotics can also be purchased over the counter. They are relatively easy to adapt to and have a high compliance among athlefes. Care must be taken in not using a "cure for all" orthotic that may treat more than one condition, thus predisposing the normal foot structures.

Hard Orthotics

Sometimes more difficult to get accustomed to initially, these devices are usually custom fit for the individual condition, but some over-the-counter varieties exist. They hold up well and are often the key to solving the mystery of pain within the kinetic chain of the body. They should be used only in patients involved in straight ahead running.

Semi-rigid Orthotics

These devices attempt to provide the support of hard orthotics but are designed to balance the feet of athletes involved in agility sports. Since each sport has its own skill requirements, the orthotic selected must reflect these differences.

Sorbothance Insoles

Sorbothane is often used to decrease impact forces. These insoles are easy to use and do not attempt to correct or alter foot mechanics.

Heel Cups

Soft heel cups are well recommended to the athlete with a "heel bruise" or "heel pain" when other possibilities have been ruled out. They help to decrease impact and to improve the shock absorption capabilities of the fat pad of the calcaneus.

Metatarsal and Longitudinal Arch Pads

Metatarsal and longitudinal arch pads, when applied to the footwear and not the foot, provide very good support to the ligamentous, bony, and muscular structures that help to form the arches of the feet and also provide some symptomatic relief for painful foot conditions. They can also be applied directly to the skin, following the previously mentioned principles of taping.

Steel Shoe Inserts

These can be used to help manage metatarsal fractures and turftoe, and in certain brands of football turf shoes are standard equipment as they are incorporated directly into the insole linear.

Conclusion

The need for research and development in the area of external support of athletic injuries is quite evident. Until such rigorous studies are conclusive, selection of taping and bracing will continue to depend on anecdotal information. Being aware of what is available, keeping abreast of new developments and analysing them carefully, and talking to others who have experience in their use can assist the sports medicine practitioner in selecting a method of support. Taping and bracing can decrease the risk of reinjury, especially when performed under the supervision of one skilled and knowledgeable in there methods. Because of the inherent nature of sport, it is paramount that the practitioner imply no guarantees.